Whispers of
Medicine's Past

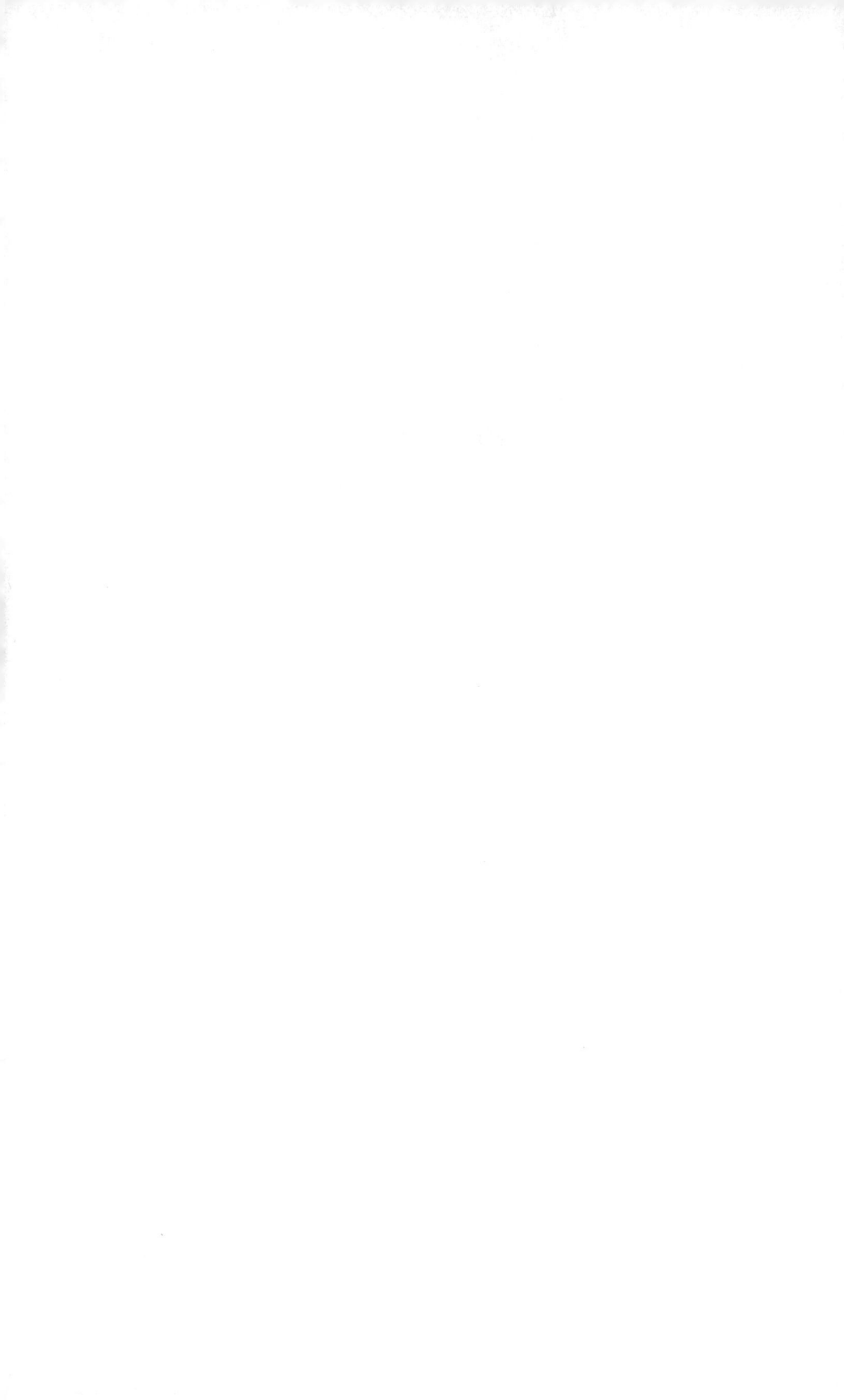

Whispers of Medicine's Past

UNEARTHING BRIGHT AND DARK TALES

Amer Husseini, MD

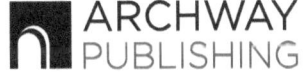

ARCHWAY
PUBLISHING

Archway Publishing books may be ordered through booksellers or by contacting:

Archway Publishing
1663 Liberty Drive
Bloomington, IN 47403
www.archwaypublishing.com
844-669-3957

ISBN: 978-1-6657-4587-1 (sc)
ISBN: 978-1-6657-4585-7 (hc)
ISBN: 978-1-6657-4586-4 (e)

Library of Congress Control Number: 2023911554

Print information available on the last page.

Archway Publishing rev. date: 09/15/2023

To my present and future grandchildren

INTRODUCTION

It requires more than good fortune for discoveries to become beneficial for humans in their daily lives.

For the process to be successful, Intellect, perseverance, and vivid imagination are all essential.

A Similar observation could pass without recognizing its significance to others until a discoverer with a vivid imagination recognizes its practical application to daily life.

Also, recognizing a potential solution to daily problems alone without perseverance would not lead to a new discovery, as many pioneers to be abandon their attempt at their first setback before achieving the glory of belonging to the Discoverer Club.

A typical example is Michael Heidelberger, and Walter Jacobs, who synthesized sulfanilamide in 1915.

Their investigation was terminated because the researchers were unable to envision that sulfonamide would be effective against bacterial infection. As a result, the development of sulfa drugs was delayed for twenty years.

The Oxford Dictionary defines Serendipity as "the faculty of making happy and unexpected discoveries by accident." It is a better word for describing the role of chance in medical discoveries because it emphasizes the role of the researcher in the process, who had to recognize the significance of the phenomenon, test it, and act on it.

Society tends to elevate researchers morally above the rest, and stories of medical breakthroughs are frequently told in a utopian style.

This book tells stories of the process of discoveries, not only its success but its setbacks,* and more importantly highlights its collateral damage, often the weak and vulnerable.

This book also uncovers some of those researchers' darker side, jealousy, backstabbing, plain racism, and in one case, alleged murder.

Finally, it revealed the poor moral standards of a society willing to put human subjects through extreme risks in the name of scientific research. Often mentally challenged children who could not have given any consent, certainly not informed one.

CHAPTER 1

ANTIBIOTICS

Alexander Gordon of Aberdeen, Scotland, was believed to be the first to suggest that puerperal (childbed) Fever was due to contamination.

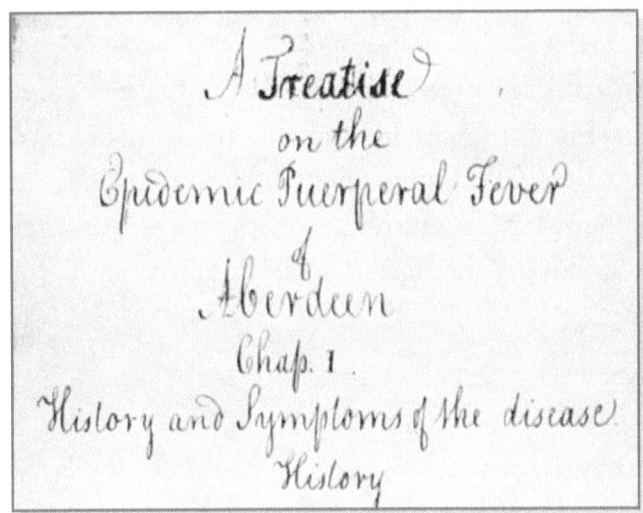

Treatise published in 1795.

In his Treatise published in 1795, he wrote a confession.

"It is a disagreeable declaration for me to mention that I was the means of carrying the infection to many women."

In the seventeenth and eighteenth centuries, Bad air or 'miasma' was thought to be associated with spreading diseases; this was a popular explanation for spreading illness in overcrowded areas, jails, ships, and warehouses.

Alexander Gordon practiced medicine in a novel way; it was what we call today "evidence base practice".

The most challenging problem for an obstetrician at the time was (Childbed) fever.

In studying the matter, he noticed that mothers living in villages Were more likely to be affected by the disease if they were cared for, by midwives from the city with prior exposure to the disease.

So, he created a table to document his theory, with the names of midwives and all deliveries they attended.

He quickly noticed that the fever happened immediately after a visit to the mother by a particular midwife. That midwife was the carrier of the disease.

That led him to recommend a Sanitation procedure to the medical community without knowing the fever's true cause.

Oliver Wendell Holmes entered Harvard in 1829 and studied law for a year before turning to medicine; he was a member of a discussion group, the Boston Society of medical improvement.

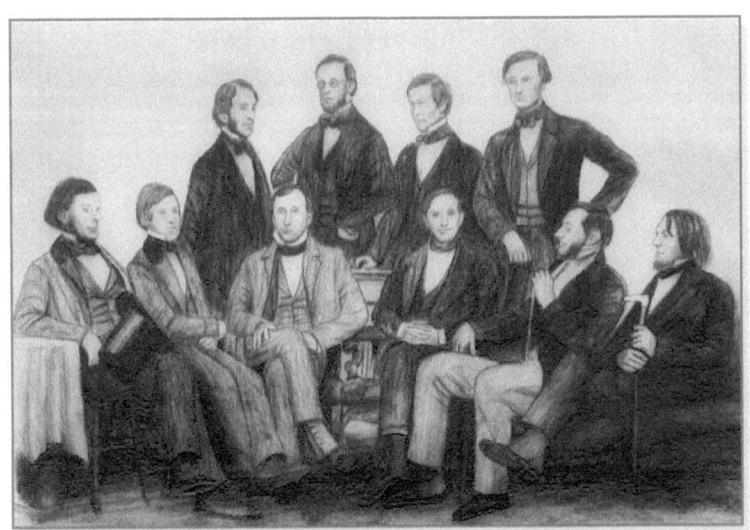

Boston Society for Medical Improvement 1853

In 1842 several cases of puerperal (Childbed) fever were reported in one of their meetings, including that of a physician, who died after sustaining the disease during an autopsy.

Doctor Holmes took it upon himself to investigate the nature of this condition, despite the fact he was not an obstetrician, and in February 1843, he presented his findings.

He concluded.

"It is the duty of the physician to take every precaution that nurses or other assistants shall not introduce the disease by making proper inquiries concerning them and giving timely warning of every suspected source of danger".

His fellow physicians attacked him, and despite the hostile receptions, he republished his article in 1855 under a different title, "Puerperal Fever as a Private Pestilence."

A few years later, in 1847, A German-Hungarian obstetrician Ignaz Semmelweis practicing in Vienna, became interested in a strange phenomenon happening across town.

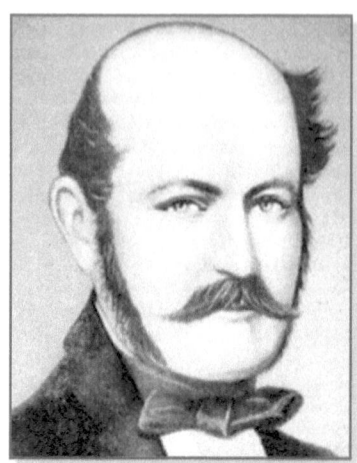

Ignaz Semmelweis

Two clinics provided free care for indigent mothers-to-be and newborns; each clinic admitted patients on an alternate day.

Still, women were begging to be admitted to the second clinic since the first clinic had a bad reputation. It had a much higher mortality rate, to the point that some women preferred to give birth in the streets, hoping to be admitted and have their child cared for in the second clinic.

His interest grew when his colleague, a pathologist, Jakob Kolletschka, had fallen ill and died after accidentally pricking his finger during an autopsy of a woman who had just died of (Childbed) fever.

Semmelweis excluded overcrowding as a cause for the higher death rate in the first clinic since the second clinic was more overcrowded and had a lower mortality rate.

Next, he noted that In the Second clinic, women gave birth on their sides, whereas in the first clinic, they gave birth on their backs. To eliminate that as the cause of the disease, he had women change positions without any change in the incidence of the death rate.

Another difference between the two clinics was that a priest was strolling past the woman's bed ringing a bell in the first clinic with the higher mortality rate; he wondered whether that experience terrified the women and caused them to have a fever and get sick, so to exclude that possibility, Semmelweis had the priest do the Same thing in the other clinic without any changes in mortality rate.

Finally, he was able to document a significant difference between the two clinics since the childbirths in clinic number one with the higher mortality were conducted by physicians and medical students; on the other hand, in the second clinic with lower mortality, midwives conducted it.

And the major difference between the practice of physicians and midwives was that the physicians and medical students were attending to the pregnant women after finishing their work in the autopsy's lab. So Semmelweis hypothesized that the students and physicians transmitted cadaverous particles to their patients.

He also hypothesized that childbed fever was affecting women in childbirth and other people in the hospital, like his colleague, the pathologist.

He chose a chlorinated lime solution to solve the problem because it was being used to eliminate the bad odor after performing autopsies, thinking that the odor was due to the cadaver's particles.

So, he demanded that all students wash their hands with the chlorinated solution before they went to help in deliveries, and the results were amazing.

The mortality rate in April 1847 was 18.3%. After hand washing was instituted in mid-May, the rates in June were 2.2 %, July 1.2 %, and August 1.9 %.

Semmelweis's theory was rejected, and some historians

attributed that rejection to the many physicians who felt they held special social status. It was inconceivable that their hands were unclean.

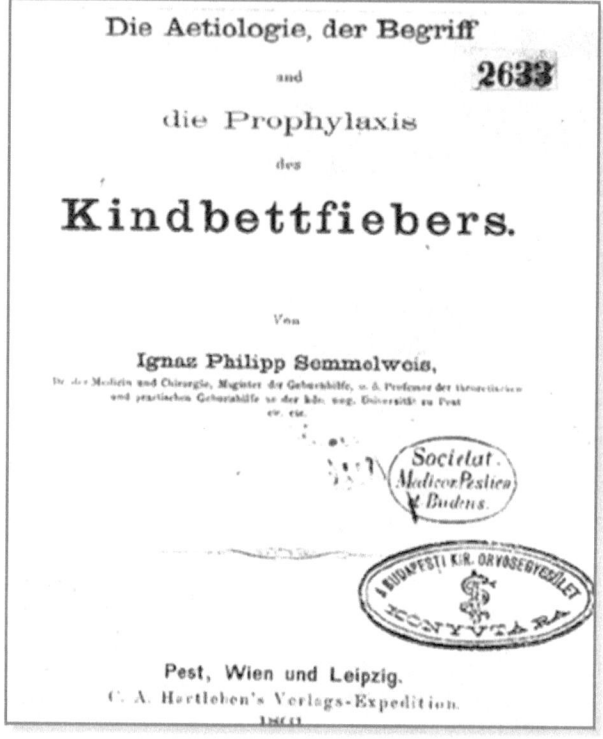

Semmelweis's article P1.4

In his 1861 book, Semmelweis wrote:

"Most medical lecture halls continue to resound with lectures on epidemic childbed fever and with discourses against my theories."

"In published medical works, my teachings are either ignored or attacked."

Unfortunately, his mental health deteriorated, and he was confined to a Mental asylum and probably beaten to death. He was 47 years old.

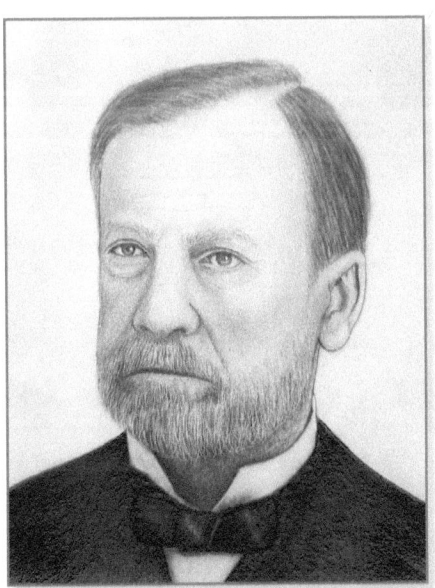

Louis pastor (1822–1895)

In 1856, A student of Louis Pasteur encouraged his father to ask Professor Pasteur to help them solve a problem; when they tried to ferment beetroot, they often did not get alcohol but acid taste fluid.

At that time, fermentation was thought to be purely a chemical reaction, but what Pasteur found was that a microscopic Organism, seen by his microscope, played a main role in converting sugar to alcohol.

Initially, he tried to boil the wine, hoping that those living particles would dissipate; unfortunately, the heat also eliminated the yeast needed for fermentation. He then tried to heat the fluid to a lower degree before fermentation and cooled it down. This process eliminated the harmful particles without affecting the useful ones. That process became known as Pasteurization.

His famous experiment disproving the theory of 'something being created from nothing' was simple but very convincing.

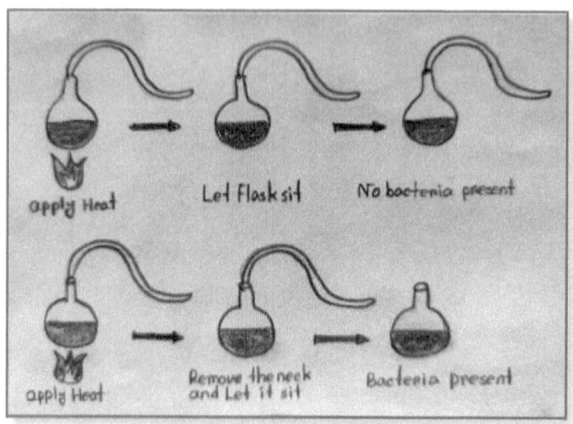

Picture of the scheme of the experimen

When boiling the fluid in the first container, which has a Swan's neck tube at its end, The fluid in the container did not have any bacteria because the bacteria carried by the dust were invisible to the naked eye and were unable to reach the fluid through the curves of that Swan's neck tube.

But when he boiled the fluid in the second container and let it sit without the Swan's neck tube, bacteria could reach the fluid, which was present when it was tested.

In 1865 Pasteur's father died, and in 1866, his two daughters were lost to typhoid fever; finally, in 1868, he suffered a stroke that kept him paralyzed on the left side, and later he died from multiple strokes.

The affinity of the dye to the fabric depends on the chemical composition of both the fabric and the dye.

Azo dye was a popular synthetic dye used in the 19th century.

In 1909 Heinrich Hoerleina, a German, while trying to improve the quality of the Azo dye, added a molecule (sulfa base) to improve its adherence to wool and patented that substance without knowing its effect on microbes.

Two American immunologists, Jacob and Heidelberger, at

Rockefeller University, synthesized sulphonamide (the same substance) in 1915 but failed to recognize its benefit; later, in 1972, Heidelberger Wrote:

"As slaves to an idea, we missed the boat in 1915, losing the chance to save many thousands of lives, and the development of the sulfonamides was delayed twenty years."

At the pharmaceutical division of I.G. Farbenindustrie, a German conglomerate, Gerhard Domagk was hired as head of scientific research by Heinrich Hoerleina, who was researching improving the quality of the Azo dye.

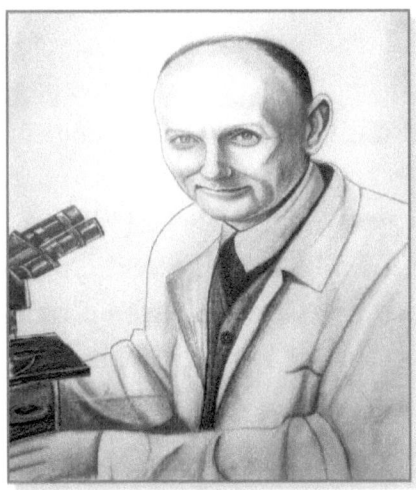

Gerhard Domagk

Domagk theorized that drug testing should be done on living creatures, even if it fails in the lab, a new approach to medical discovery and research.

His main assignment was to identify agents to combat common infectious diseases.

Domagk used infected mice to test several compounds, like gold and acridine dyes, and the results were disappointing.

However, in the 1930s, the results were better and more

encouraging, as compound KL 695 was synthesized, although it was ineffective in lab tubes; it was found to have a weak effectiveness property in infected mice, later another compound KL 730 was discovered, which had a remarkable benefit.

He tested 26 infected mice. Fourteen as controls, and twelve were injected with a large dose of the red dye; all mice in the control group died within a few days, while all the treated mice survived.

That dye was named Prontosil rubrum, and the medication was patented as Prontosil, the first widely used (sulfa) antibiotic.

Three years have passed since Prontosil was synthesized till the initial clinical report was published; Domagk's Defenders Claimed that the reason was his dedication to efficacy and safety. His opponents claimed that the company wanted to keep the results secret until the drug patent problems were resolved.

During those three years, Domagk treated many people, including his six-year-old daughter, Hildegard, who had contracted an infection from a needle, with Prontosil. Luckily, she recovered; however, the treatment left a permanent reddish discoloration of her skin due to the dye, which became the drug.

Prontosil (sulfa) was not accepted immediately, but in 1935, an unexpected and lucky event changed the tide.

Eleanor Roosevelt missed the family Thanksgiving dinner to be next to her son, who was in Boston suffering from a Septic sore throat. His doctor treated him successfully with the sulfa drug (Prontosil), that incident was reported in the popular press, including the New York Times, with an announcement like this.

"A new control for infections had been discovered."

Prontosil, a dye, was hard to dissolve to prepare in a liquid form for children's consumption; in 1937, a small company in Bristol, Tennessee tried to do that. Unfortunately, and unknowingly they used a toxic chemical as a solvent. Without any testing, the elixir was distributed to the public, and 108 people, mostly children, died from kidney and liver failure.

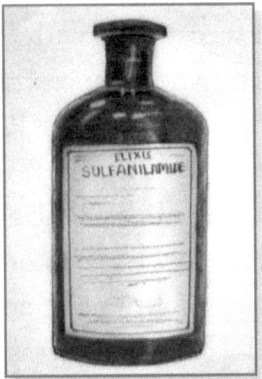

Sulfanamide elixir P 1.8

Unfortunately, due to a lack of regulation, the company paid a fine of merely $16,000; however, the chemist behind this project committed suicide two years later.

Despite this tragedy, Prontosil use expanded Between 1940 and 1942 because of the war, sulfur powder and sulfur tablets were part of the combat medic's kit.

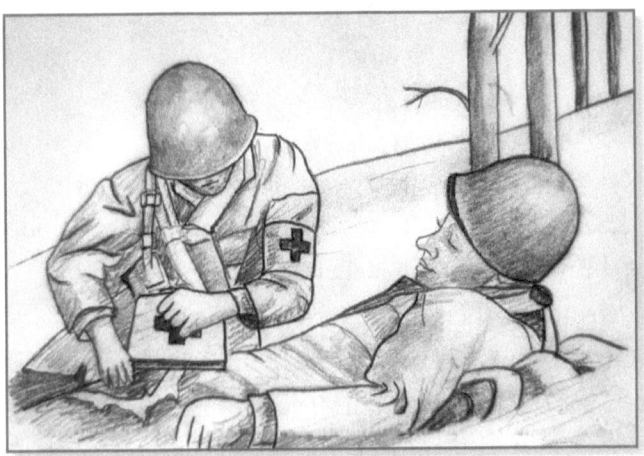

Soldiers in WWII

After attending the Tehran conference in 1943, on his way home, Winston Churchill's airplane, a York transport Ascalon, landed in Tunisia urgently because he was suffering from pneumonia; he was treated successfully with a sulfa compound.

Meanwhile, the British newspapers mistakenly declared that Penicillin, a British invention, was the Prime Minister's savior, and the story became a legend, but it was untrue.

Dr John Mather, Churchill's physician, wrote:

"A fundamental problem with the story is that Churchill was treated for this severe strain of pneumonia not with Penicillin but with M&B ", a sulfa drug which was a German invention.

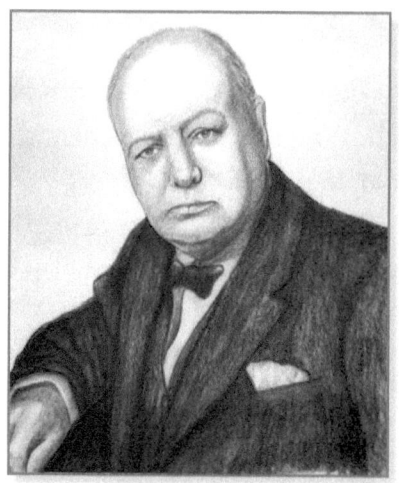

Winston Churchill

IN 1939 Gerhard Domagk was awarded the Nobel prize; initially, he wrote a letter accepting the prize, but two weeks later, he wrote another letter "rather regretfully declined" Under pressure from the Gestapo, after spending a week in jail.

Later, in 1947 he was able to reclaim the gold medal and the diploma, but he could no longer receive the $35,000 prize money.

Alexander Fleming returned from his vacation To Saint Mary's Hospital in London on September 3rd, 1928, to find one of his bacterial containers was different from the other; a Fungus was growing in this sample container and was preventing the bacteria from growing; he called the fungus penicillin.

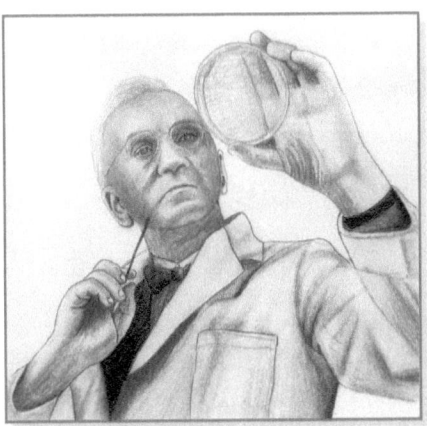

Alexander Fleming P1.11

He published his finding in 1929 without any comment about Penicillin's potential benefit in treating infection, and ironically, he did very little work on Penicillin afterward because he did not have enough help at Saint Mary's hospital.

The Oxford group consisted of Howard Florey, Ernst Chain, and others who worked on purifying and producing Penicillin. They were partially successful.

In May 1939, they infected eight mice with Strep Bacteria; after that, they injected four of them with Penicillin, and the other four were used as an untreated control group.

The result was described as a "miracle," as all mice in the control group died, and all treated ones survived.

In 1941, the Oxford team produced a decent amount of Penicillin; they decided to test it on humans.

In 1941, Albert Alexander, 48, an Oxford police constable, was suffering from severe infection with Abscess formation in his face failed sulfa treatment and became the ideal candidate to be treated with Penicillin, the experimental drug at the time.

Although he got much better initially, as the story said, he died a few weeks later, because the investigator run out of penicillin.

A year later, on March 14, 1942, Anne Miller, who was dying from streptococcal septicemia, was treated with Penicillin. She fully recovered and became the first patient cured with Penicillin.

Florey and Heatley recognized their inability to produce a satisfactory amount of Penicillin, so they traveled in the summer of 1941 to Peoria, IL, in the United States to try to convince pharmaceutical companies to join the effort in producing Penicillin.

By chance, Mary Hunt, a laboratory assistant, brought a rotten melon covered with golden mold that turned out to have 200 times the yield of Penicillin from the species Fleming isolated.

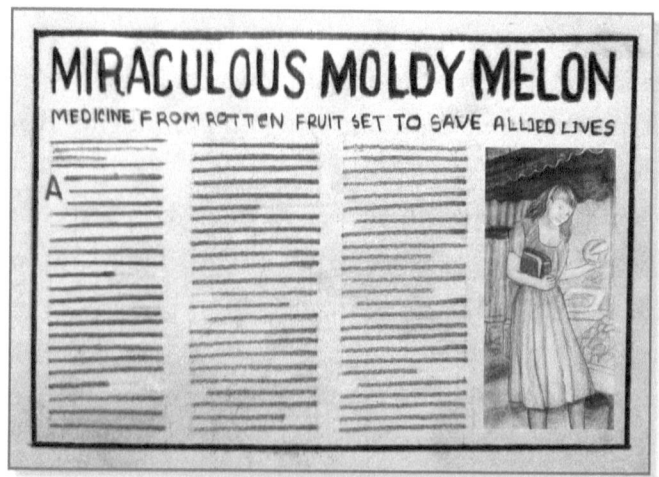

Mary Hunt in the news

Penicillin was never patented because it was a natural product, but the production method had a patent number of US 2442141A.

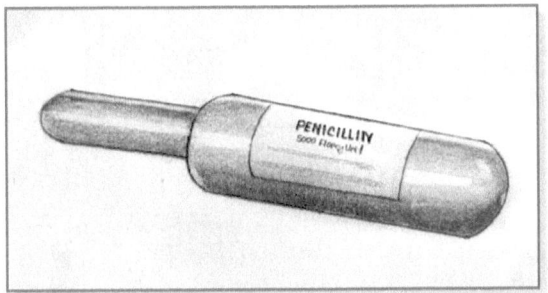

Penicillin ampule

Initially, Fleming was credited alone for the discovery of Penicillin, but later in 1945, the Nobel Prize committee awarded its prize correctly to Fleming, Florida, and Chain (Oxford group)

CHAPTER 2

ASPIRIN

The ancient world did not know Aspirin; however, Willow bark was used to treat nonspecific pain.

Edwin Smith bought two ancient documents in 1862 in Cairo; they dated back to 1500 BC, one of them is known as Ebers papyrus Which records over 150 remedies; one of those treatments was the white willow bark.

Both Hippocrates (460 -377 BC) and Galen (130-200 AD) Recommended chewing Willow bark, which contains a similar chemical material to Aspirin, for their patients.

In 1828, Joseph Buchner, a pharmacist in Munich, produced a bitter-tasting yellow crystal that he named 'salicin', after salix, the Latin name for willow.

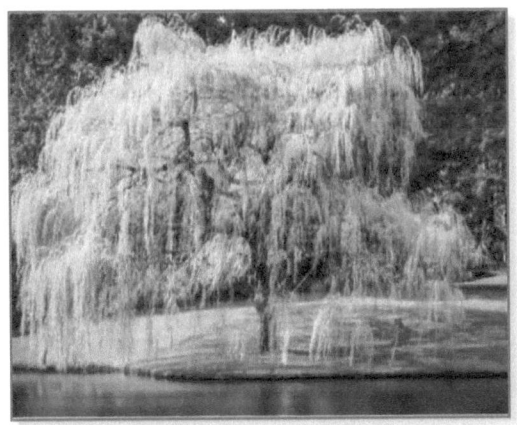

The willow tree's bark is the source of "salicin."

In 1876, Thomas MacLagan, a Scotch physician, took Salicin to monitor its effect on his own body before giving it to his patients.

'I determined to give salicin; but before doing so, took myself first five, then ten, then thirty grains without experiencing the least inconvenience or discomfort'.

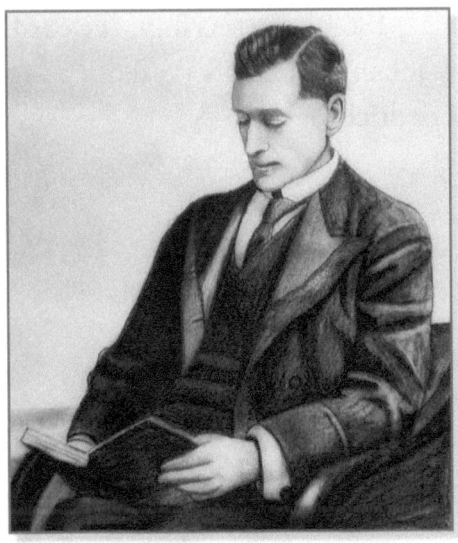

Thomas MacLagan

MacLagan treated eight patients with Rheumatic fever and reported improvement in their symptoms.

Before the treatment, the patient's temperature Was recorded between 101.8° and 103° F, with a pulse of 120 beats per minute and swollen and painful joints.

One day after the Salicin was started. The patient's temperature came down to 99.6 Fahrenheit, and his pulse reached 100; his swollen and painful joints also improved.

In the Lancet, Maclagan wrote:

"The sudden arrest of the painful symptoms, and the coincident rapid fall of pulse and temperature, followed so immediately on the administration of the Salicin that it is impossible not to attribute them to its use. Cases of acute rheumatism do sometimes improve most unexpectedly, but I never saw a case get well so quickly as I have given the details above. A succession of such cases cannot but be attributed to the peculiarity of the treatment."

Despite that success, Salicin did not become popular because of its side effect on the stomach.

On August 1st, 1863, a partnership, "Friedr Bayer et comp," was founded by Johann Friedrich Weskott, a master dyer and a dye salesman Friedrich Bayer.

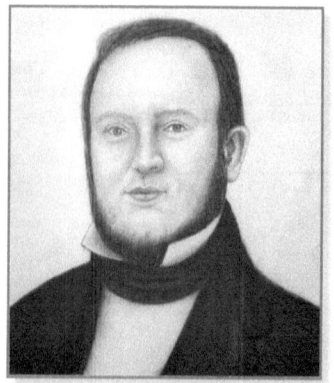
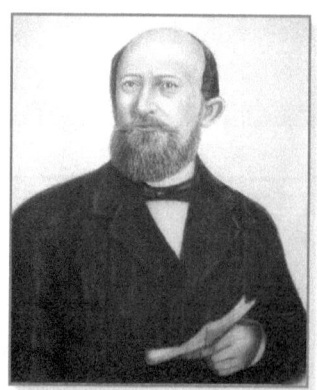

Johann Friedrich Weskott   *Friedrich Bayer*

The company was to manufacture and sell synthetic dye-stuffs since, before that, only natural dye was used in the textile industry, because natural dye was expensive and scarce.

Their experience in dealing with chemicals grew because of the nature of their business, and the pharmaceutical field was their next area of expansion Opportunity.

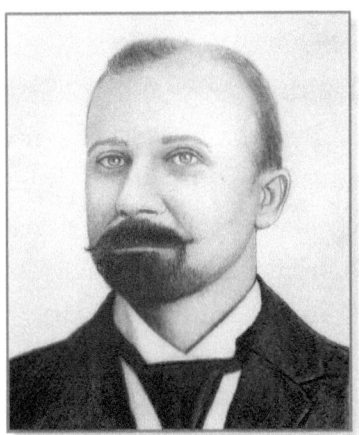

Felix Hoffmann
inventor of Aspirin and Heroin

Felix Hoffman's father was suffering from rheumatic disease, and he influenced his son to discover Aspirin to avoid a side effect of sodium salicylates.

Hoffmann (1868–1946) was a chemist working since graduation in 1893 for "Friedr Bayer et comp "in the newly established pharmaceutical research department. His colleagues thought that Hoffman had a "good nose" for discovery.

In the summer of 1897, Hoffmann added the acetyl group (CH_3CO) to all sorts of molecules; since "acetylating" molecules had worked with Bayer's earlier medications, the result was the first sample of pure acetylsalicylic acid (Aspirin) on 10 August 1897

Initially, Heinrich Dreser, the head of Bayer's pharmaceutical laboratory, dismissed the new product and declared ("The product has no value") on the ground that it has a side effect on the heart and causes palpitation; some historians believed the real reason for his refusal was his enthusiastic support to Heroin, which Phillips Hoffman himself invented.

Another executive at Bayer, Arthur Eichengruen (whose job was to originate new products), refused to accept Dreser's rejection of acetylsalicylic acid; eventually, Dreser changed his mind and tested Aspirin on himself.

While Hoffmann and Eichengrün did not receive any royalties for the development of Aspirin, only Dreser was paid royalties and went on to make a fortune from the development of Aspirin.

Eichengrün's contribution to the discovery was neglected, and he could not claim his role in the discovery because Eichengrün was a Jewish. In 1944; he was sent to the Theresienstadt concentration camp, where he remained until the Russians liberated it in 1945.

It was not until 1949, 15 years after Hoffmann's discovery, Arthur Eichengrün published an article claiming that the discovery was made under his direction.

Acetylsalicylic acid was given the name Aspirin from the A for acetyl and the Spirin from Spirea, the name of shrubs that was a salicylic acid source.

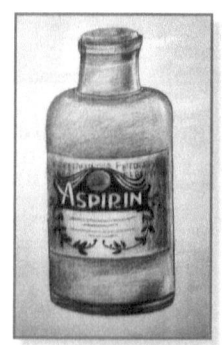

Earlier Aspirin in a powder form

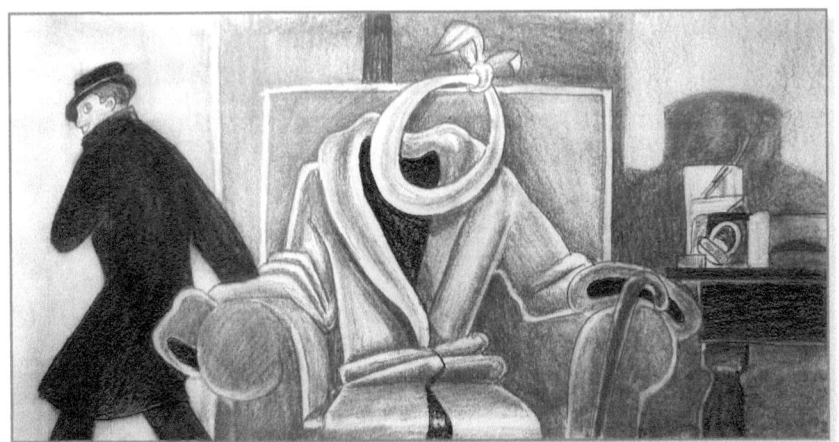

An early advertisement for Bayer aspirin.

A not well-known, average family physician, Lawrence Craven in California, recorded an observation in a regional medical journal in 1950.

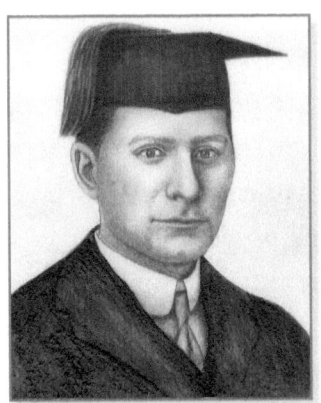

Dr Lawrence Craven

Dr Graven wrote:

"For 36 years, my surgical work has been primarily the removal of tonsils and adenoids. Of the hundreds of cases handled, only five were performed in hospitals. Surgery was performed during morning office hours, and practically all patients were released to their homes by early afternoon without question of possible hemorrhage—practically none occurred until about six years ago. At which time, an alarming number of hemorrhages were evidenced in disturbing frequency."

Craven attributed the increased bleeding complications to a new medicine, aspirin gum, which was being given to relieve pain.

He took Aspirin to experiment on himself, and in 1950 he wrote.

"Ingestion of 12 aspirin tablets daily resulted in spontaneous profuse nosebleed after five days. In order to check on the reliability of this observation, the test was repeated twice over, with precisely the same results. The proof seemed all the more convincing as the author had not experienced a nosebleed for more than fifty years."

Knowing that heart attacks were due to blood clots, Doctor Craven recommended his male patient between the ages of 45 and 65 take Aspirin to prevent heart attacks. He followed 400 of these patients for two years; later, he reported no single heart attack among those patients.

He continued his observation, and his final count was up to about 8,000 patients; only nine of them died of what they thought was due to a heart attack; however, the autopsy proved that it was a ruptured aorta.

Since it was observational without any controlled group, his study was dismissed by the medical community and was forgotten.

The continuing use of Aspirin increased the incidents of bleeding, visible or overt, which prompted many scientists to explore the possibility that aspirin effect coagulations.

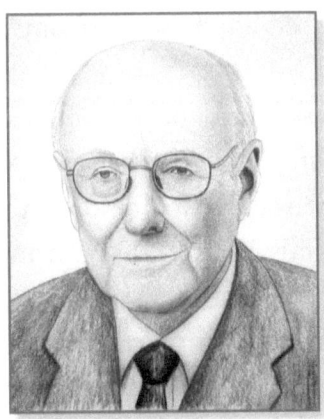

Dr Harvey J. Weiss

Sometime in 1971 or 1972, Dr. Harvey J. Weiss, a hematologist from New York, gave a talk in Ann Arbor, Michigan, on platelet disorders; at the end of his talk, he mentioned that Aspirin has a beneficial potential in treating arterial thrombosis.

On the way back home, he shared a cab with a physician going to the airport; that physician told Dr Weiss that he had read an article regarding Aspirin's effect in preventing heart attack, published decades earlier, and he did not remember the author's name or the name of the journal. Still, he said that it was 'some Southern journal.'

The hospital's librarian found that the article was published in the Mississippi Valley Medical Journal in 1953. It was Lawrence Craven's Article.

The "Southern" journal was published in Quincy, Illinois, about 100 miles west of Abraham Lincoln's home.

Dr Weiss experimented on dogs to study the effect of aspirin on platelets' functions and thrombosis [clotting].

He injured the common carotid or femoral artery, either by mechanical or chemical means, and measured the degree of thrombosis induced in these segments, with and without Aspirin.

Aspirin reduced the incidence of total occlusion significantly, although it didn't completely prevent that phenomenon.

Later a One thousand two hundred thirty-nine men discharged from hospitals in the UK with myocardial infarction [heart attack] were enrolled in a study. Participants were given either Aspirin 300 mg daily or a matching gelatin capsule.

While fewer participants treated with Aspirin died six months later, the difference was not statistically significant, and the trial was considered inconclusive.

Not until another large trial called "the Second International Study of Infarct Survival (ISIS-2)", aspirin benefits were proven. This trial was conducted between March 1985 and December 1987 to study the efficacy of Aspirin in patients with an acute heart attack.

This study enrolled 17,187 patients from 417 hospitals within 24 hours after the onset of suspected acute Heart Attack. Aspirin use significantly reduced non-fatal reinfarction, stroke, vascular mortality, and all-cause mortality.

Aspirin became one of the main drugs, used in treating heart disease.

CHAPTER

BLOOD TRANSFUSION

In 1492, Pope Innocent VIII became ill and lastly unconscious. Hence, his physician Giacomo di San recommended treating the Pope with the blood of three young boys to resuscitate him by making the Pope swallow the blood. The story is not entirely reliable and might have been an Anti-Semitic fabrication because the physician was Jewish.

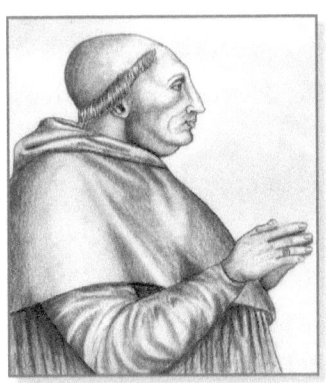

Pope Innocent VIII

Richard Lower, a physician at Oxford, attempted to transfuse wine, milk, and broth to animals. Finally, in 1665, he transfused a small amount of blood between two dogs without any benefit or ill effect.

Two years later, in 1667, French physician Jean-Baptiste Denys recorded the first blood transfusion from animal to human after many successful attempts to transfuse blood from animal to animal.

Denys Elected to use animals' blood on moral grounds:

"It barbarous to shorten the life of one man to extend the life of another."

His first patient was a 15-year boy who lost a significant amount of blood during leeching by another physician; Denys transfused an insignificant amount of sheep's blood (12 oz). The treatment was declared a huge success, but retrospectively, the amount of blood transfused was minimal to have any benefits.

However, his third patient, a Swedish royal called Gustaf Bonde, was not as lucky, as he died after his second transfusion.

That bad experience did not stop Denys from trying again, and his victim was a mentally ill man Antoine Mauroy, who did not survive his third transfusion.

Denys was sued by the man's wife for killing her husband.

Denys produced a witness to testify that a cat died after eating the spoiled food which Mrs. Mauroy used to feed her husband.

Dr Denys was exonerated, and it was reported that Mrs. Mauroy was convicted of killing her husband using arsenic, she was hanged. As a result of the fiasco, the French Parliament prohibited blood transfusions.

Across the channel, in Cambridge, England, Richard Lower, in the same year (1667), transfused the blood of a lamb to Arthur

Coga, an educated 32-year-old man whose brain was described as "was sometimes a little too warm" thinking that the lamb blood would cool his brain.

The poor patient declared in Latin, 'Sanguis ovis symbolicam quandam facul-tatem habet cum sanguine Christi, quia Christus est Agnus Dei' ('the blood of sheep has symbolic power like the blood of Christ, for Christ is the Lamb of God').

Coga changed his mind and said the blood transfusion turned him into a sheep, and he was lucky to survive. However, another patient's death prompted outlawing of blood transfusion in England as a result of transfusing the blood of a lamb.

In 1799, Dr William Thornton believed a transfusion would resurrect his friend, President George Washington, by blood transfusion.

Dr Thornton never stopped believing that blood transfusion could infuse life into a human, thinking that blood is the source of life.

He wrote two decades later: "There was no doubt in my mind that his restoration was possible."

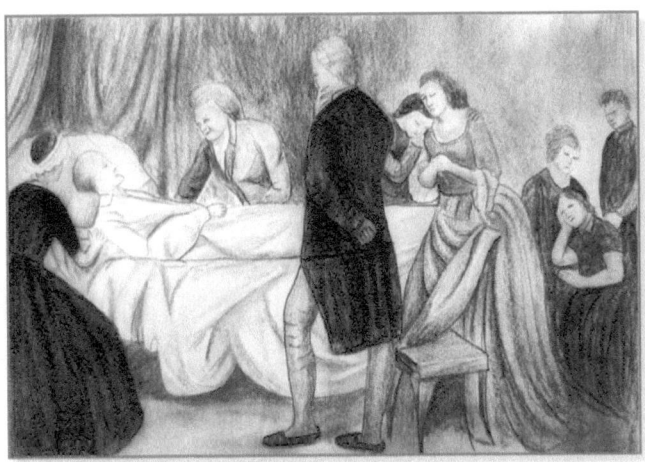

President Washington on his Deathbed

British obstetrician James Blundell conducted experimental transfusion on animals in the early nineteenth century. He found out that after bleeding a dog almost to death, he was able to save the dog with a blood transfusion from another dog. This process failed when he transfused the dying dog with sheep's blood.

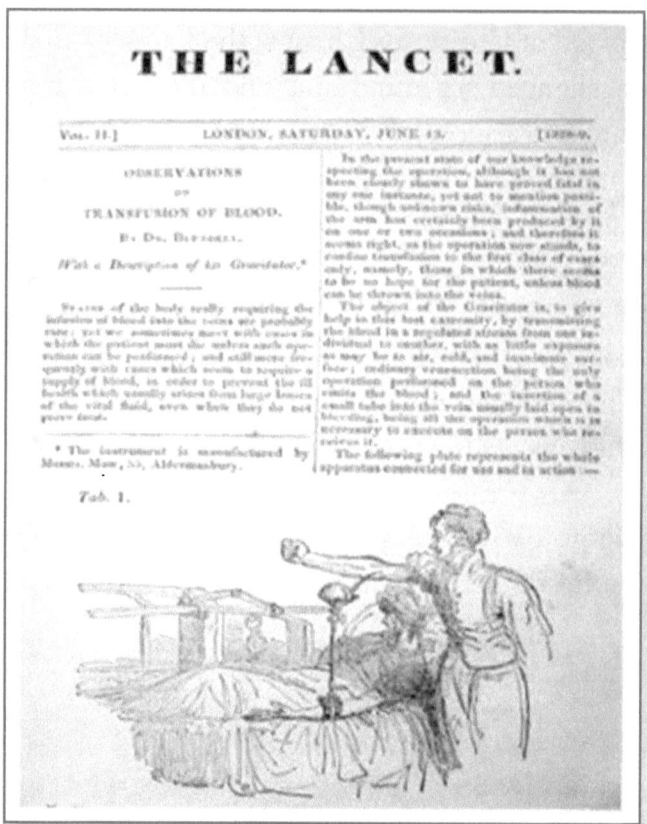

Lancet publication

In 1818 James Blundell transfused the blood of a husband to his dying wife, who bled profusely after delivery,with success and reported later in 1928 in the Lancet his experience with ten more patients; some were successful, others were not.

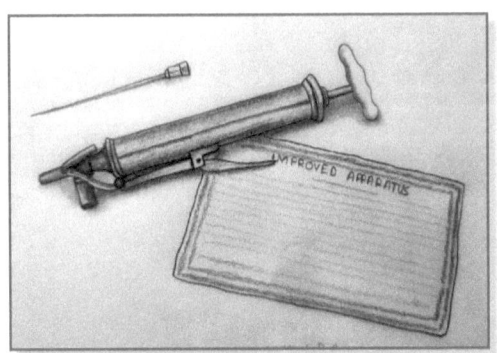

Blundell's transfusion kit.

In 1854, Drs James Bovel and Edwin Holder from Toronto, Canada, believed that particles in milk would eventually be transformed into "white corpuscles," or white blood cells.

They transfused a 40-year-old man 12 ounces of cow's milk. The patient seemed to respond to the treatment well. They tried again with success. They tried five times again, but all their patients died.

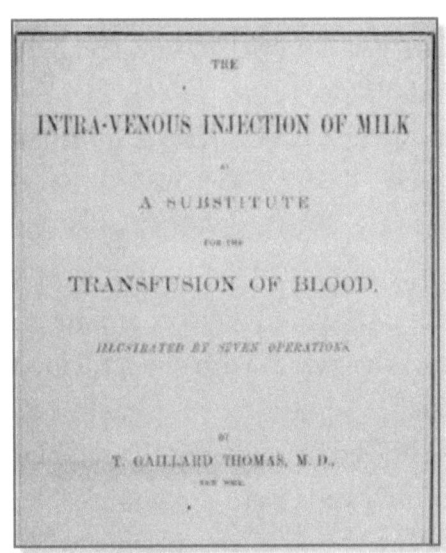

Milk Transfusion
A publication by T. Gaillard 1832-1903

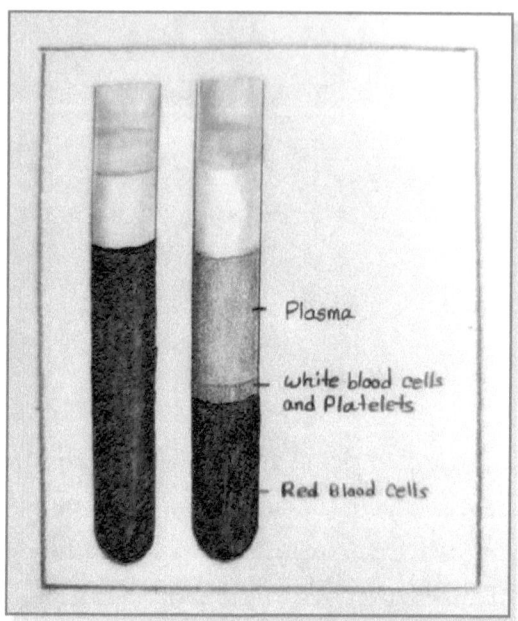

Blood components

When blood is left in a laboratory tube, it separates into three components: the red blood cells at the bottom, the white blood cells and platelets just above that, and finally, the plasma, the yellow clear fluid on top.

In 1900, at the age of 32, Karl Landsteiner, an Austrian physician, was puzzled why some blood transfusion between the same species was successful and others were not.

He studied the sample blood of four people, his colleague and himself, a total of six individuals, and he mixed the plasma (the liquid part of the blood) with the red blood cells from different individuals.

Some tubes showed clumping of the red blood cells because the plasma and their cells were not compatible; others did not show the clumping, because the plasma with the cells were compatible.

T a b e l l e III, betreffend das Blut von fünf Puerperae und sechs Placenten (Nabelschnurblut).

Sera	Trautm.	Linsm.	Seil.	Freib.	Graupn.	Mittelb.
Lust.	+	+	−	−	−	+
Tomsch.	−	−	+	−	−	−
Mittelb.	−	−	+	−	−	−
Seil.	−	−	+	−	−	−
Linsm.	+	+	+	−	−	+
Blutkörperchen von:						

The reaction of mixing plasma with red cells in different individuals.

That led him to the discovery of three different blood types, groups A.B. and O.

Later, one of his students discovered a fourth type, the AB group.

Dr Landsteiner was asked what the practical use of his discovery was.

He answered:

'I think this discovery may aid in determining the perpetrator at the crime scene.'

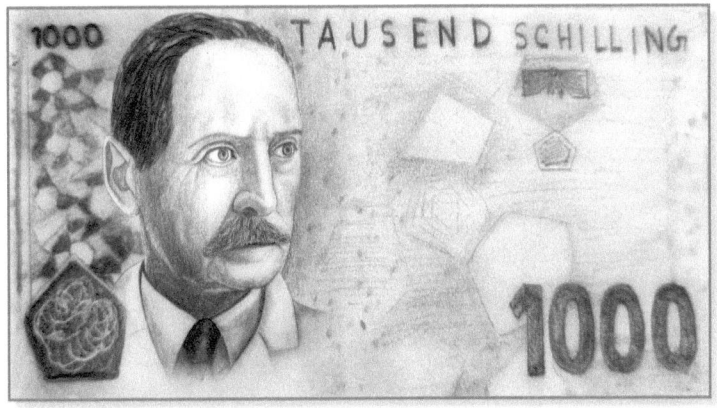

Old Austrian currency note bearing the picture of Karl Landsteiner

Although he was born in Vienna, he became an American citizen by the time he won the Nobel Prize in 1930, becoming the first US citizen to win a Nobel Prize in medicine.

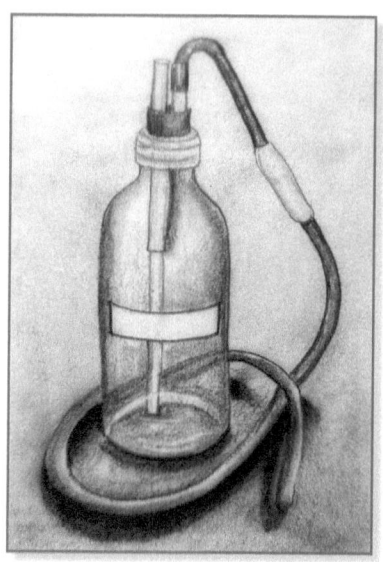

Blood transfusion apparatus used in 1907

In 1907, a New York doctor, Reuben Ottenberg, mixed up the donor's and the patient's blood to confirm compatibility and was given credit for being the first to transfuse blood successfully using the new method.

CHAPTER 4

CORONARY ANGIOGRAPHY

An old painting from the work of the French physiologist Marey, of a man introducing a catheter into a horse's heart through the horse's jugular vein, inspired a young physician, 25 years old at that time, in a small hospital outside Berlin, Germany.

Werner Forssmann wanted to use that catheter to introduce medications into the heart quickly and directly.

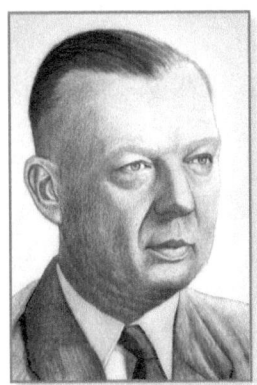

Werner Forssmann

In 1929, Forssman practiced passing a catheter into the vein and the heart on a cadaver first. His success, made him present his plan of trying it on himself to his boss, who refused to allow the experiment.

On his first attempt, his colleague, Peter Romeis, inserted a foley catheter into Forssmann's arm, but Dr Romeis panicked and stopped when he felt resistant.

A week later, Forssmann convinced Gerda Ditzen, the head nurse for the operating room, to help him in the experiment, and she volunteered to be the subject. Her cooperation was mandatory, as she kept all equipment needed locked up .

On the experiment day, she wanted to sit during the catheter insertion, but Forssmann insisted that she lay down because of the possible side effect of the anesthesia.

After preparing her arm for the incision, to her surprise, he had her hands and feet tied to the table, made the incision on his arm, and introduced the Foley catheter in his vein for 30 CM.

After that, he released her and asked that she accompany him to the x-ray machine, one story below, his friend, Peter Romeis, showed up again and tried to pull the catheter out but could not because of Forssmann's resistance.

Using a mirror to see the fluoroscopy images, Forssmann noted that the catheter was still far from the heart, so he advanced until it was 60 cm inside his body; at that time, a chest x-ray was done to document the success.

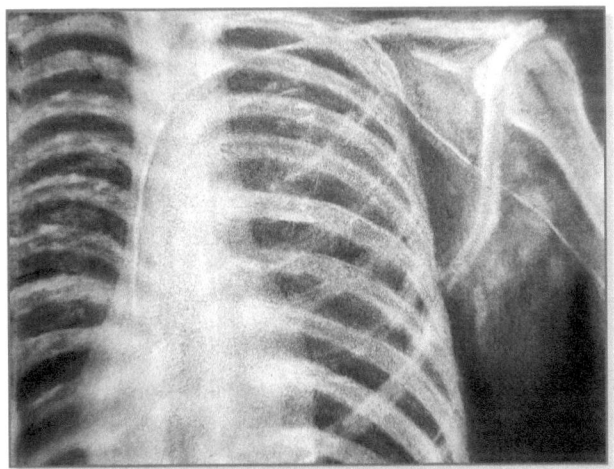

Chest x-ray with the catheter in the heart

Forssmann was granted permission to insert a Catheter in a dying woman to study the effect of direct infusion of a medication in the heart cavity directly.

After he published his article in November 1929 describing his work and discovery, many in the German medical and academic community were not supportive.

Several attempts to find research opportunities were unsuccessful, so Forssmann lost interest in cardiac catheterizing and ended up practicing urology.

Forssmann joined the Nazi party in 1932 and served in the German Army. He was later captured and spent several years as a prisoner of war in a US POW's camp. After his release in 1945, he was forbidden from medical practice and worked as a lumberjack; in 1950, he was allowed to practice urology again.

Despite his affiliation with the Nazi party, he was awarded the Noble Price in 1956 with André Cournand and Dickinson W. Richards, who developed ways to apply his technique to heart disease diagnosis in New York.

Before October 30th, 1958, there was overwhelming agreement that injecting dye into the coronary arteries would lead to death since many researchers reported a 100% fatality rate when contrast media was selectively injected into the coronary arteries of dogs.

On that day, in the Cleveland Clinic, lay a 26-year-old patient on the cardiac catheterization table; He had aortic valve disease.

Dr Mason Sones, a pediatric cardiologist, was evaluating that patient's heart in cardiac catheterization lab.

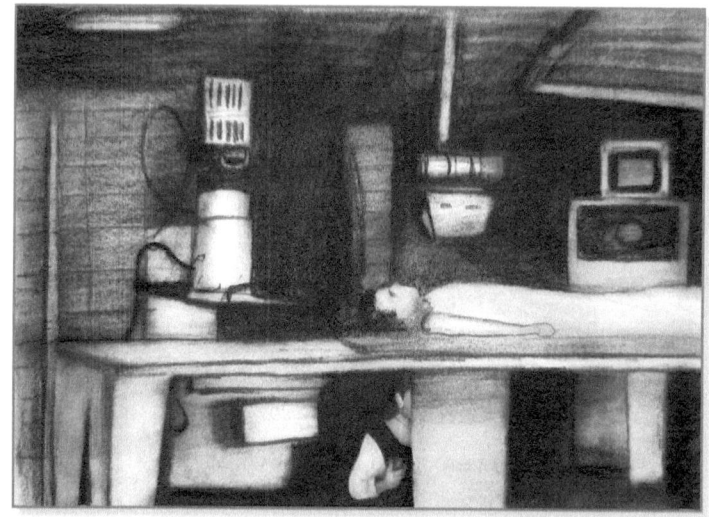

Picture of an old catheterization lab

In those days, there was Pit under that table for the operator to stand, so he could see the catheter and dye when it was injected.

The catheter was inserted inside the left ventricle of the heart, and after injecting dye, it was pulled back into the Aorta to inject more dye to take a picture of the Aorta.

Evidently, the catheter position was not verified, according to one account, and Dr. Mason gave the trainee the order to fire the injector while Mason watched from the pit.

To Mason's horror, he saw that the catheter was engaged into the right coronary artery, and all the dye was injected into that artery; he screamed, "Pull it out, we're killing him."

Mason climbed out of the pit, reached for a scalpel, to open the patient's chest, because indirect cardioversion was not discovered yet and chest compression resuscitation was not practiced yet.

To Mason's surprise, the patient did not fibrillate, but his heart stopped beating, which is a much easier problem to manage, with a combination of Atropine (a medication that increases the heart rate) and asking the patient to cough," Cough, goddamn it!". A big disaster was avoided, and a new frontier was discovered.

However, because of the absence of treatment for coronary artery disease, the procedure's value in managing patients with coronary artery disease was questioned because coronary surgery was primitive, coronary artery bypass surgery had not been invented yet, and coronary angioplasty was invented decades later.

Dr. Sones did not publish his experiment till 1962, several years after that October day; the reason for the delay was, according to several accounts, because he had dyslexia and hated writings.

His colleague Dr Proudfit in the Cleveland Clinic suggested conducting a study to find the correlation between the clinical finding by history, physical examination, EKG, and coronary angiogram, but Sones did not allow it on the first 1000 cases because he wanted to build the experience of the angiographers to get an accurate answer.

A decade after Dr. Sones' death, Dr. Proudfit said: "at first some people thought he was a nut—which he was," and continued "But they became convinced that he was a smart nut."

Dr Mason Sones was a chain smoker and used sterile forceps to hold a lit cigarette while doing coronary angiography; he died of lung cancer at the age of 66.

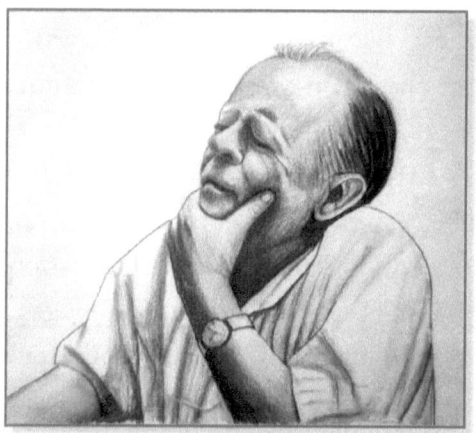

Dr F. Mason Sones

Although coronary surgeries have been performed using different techniques since 1964 with variable usefulness and success, coronary bypass surgery was also done in a sporadic instance, as a bail-out in an emergency.

But it was not until 9th May 1967 that the door for modern coronary bypass surgery was opened in the Cleveland clinic by an Argentinian surgeon of Italian heritage, Dr Rene Favaloro.

After practicing in a humble rural Argentine, Dr Favalero came to the Cleveland Clinic for training late in life.

He was 38 years; his vast experience in Argentina prepared him to excel while training at the Cleveland Clinic. Most importantly, the fact that Mason Sones discovered selective coronary angiography a few years earlier opened the door for Favarolo to be the father of coronary bypass surgery.

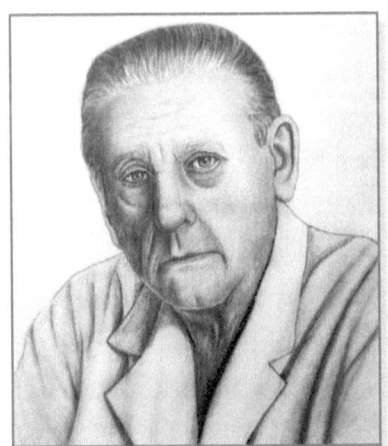

Renee Favalero

He was called the father of coronary bypass surgery, not because he did the first surgery of that kind, but because he performed that surgery systematically with acceptable risks and complications rate on a consistent basis.

In 1970, Dr Favalero decided to return to Argentina, despite a generous offer from the Cleveland clinic; according to one report, a two-million-dollar yearly salary.

Dr Favalero was able to raise enough money to build a medical teaching Foundation modeled after the Cleveland Clinic in Buenos Aires, Argentina.

Thousands of patients were treated in that foundation, and hundreds of surgeons were trained, but because of the philosophy that medicine should be available for all, his foundation ran into financial difficulties.

He is known to have said:

"I have always practiced medicine with a profound social pledge. For me, all patients are equal. Every patient, paying or not, will continue receiving the same attention!"

Dr Favalero was married for over 48 years to his wife Maria, who died in 1998; they had no children.

On July 29th, 2000, Dr Favaloro's secretary found his body in the bathroom of his apartment; he committed suicide by shooting himself in the heart; he was 77 years old.

For inventors and developers to succeed, they must use all the knowledge and experiences their predecessors left and give credit to those who inspired them.

They need to gain the support of influential people around them; if a mistake is made, they learn from it, and when a setback occurs, they have to pick up what was left and start again.

Andreas Gruentzig was one of those inventors; he was born in the eastern part of Germany and just missed the big prison created by building the iron wall; he ended up in Zurich, Switzerland.

Many contributions were made to the field of vascular disease before Dr Gruentzig.

In 1964, Mrs Laura Shaw was about to lose her leg because of a stenotic artery (blocked artery), and she refused the amputation, knowing that she could lose her life.

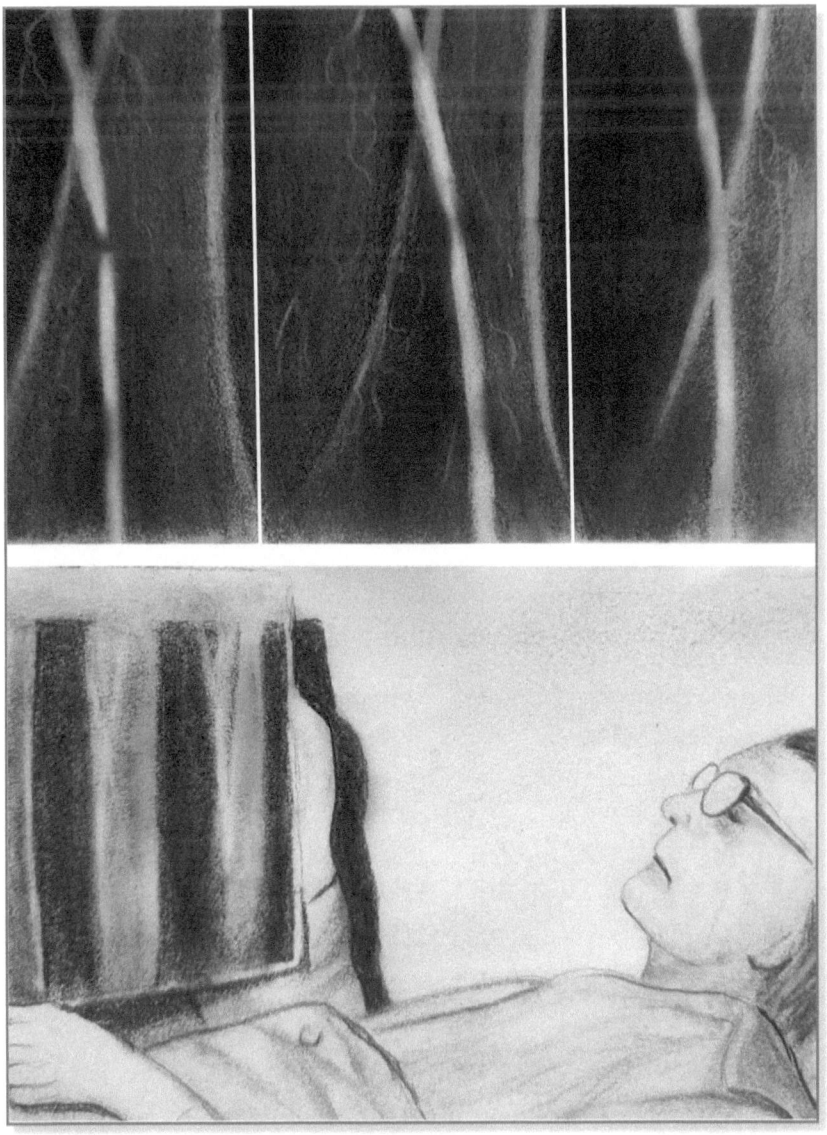

Laura Shaw

Luckily for her and us, Dr. Charles Dotter was a radiologist practicing in Portland, Oregon, at the same hospital Mrs Shaw was being treated.

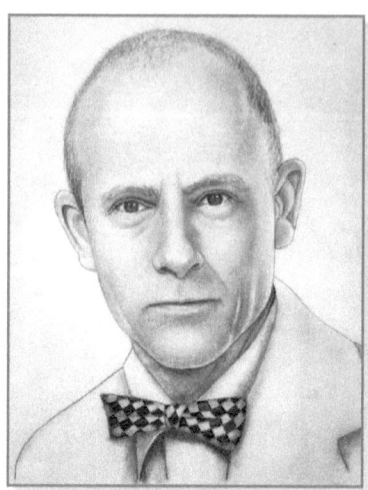

Dr Charles Dotter

Dr Dotter sled a series of catheters of successive sizes through the blocked artery in the leg till the blockage was dilated.

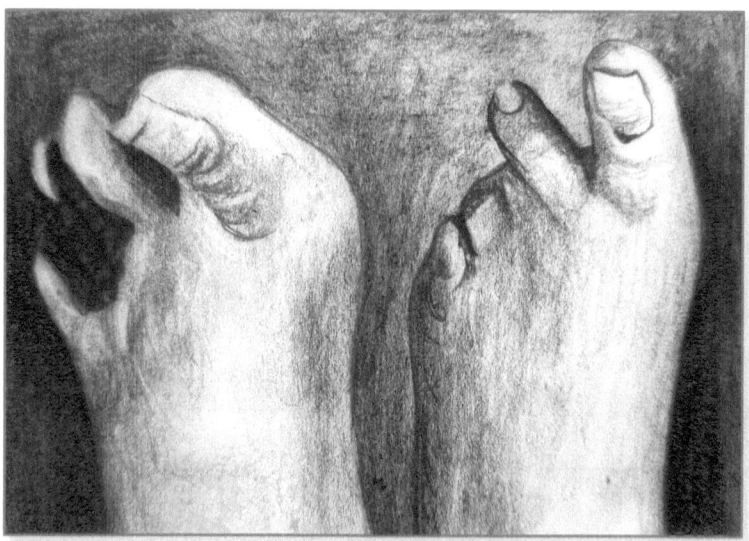

Mrs Shaw's leg ulcer healed, and she lived another three years after that, "still walking on my own two feet", as she always said.

In the late 1960s, Grüntzig found his patient's remark fascinating when the patient asked him:

Whether it was possible to just 'clean' his obstructed arteries, like a plumber.

Shortly after that, Grüntzig was introduced to Dotter's technique in dilating stenotic artery (blocked artery), but his chief warned him not to get involved.

«I will never allow this technique to be practiced at my hospital."

Using a balloon on the tip of the catheter to dilate the stenosis (blockage) was not new, and many researchers attempted to build such a catheter long before Grüntzig's success.

After working for two years at his kitchen table, trying to build a catheter with a balloon at its tip without success, a shoelaces factory provided Grundzeg with a silk mesh to wrap around the balloon to give the balloon a much-needed support.

The next step was to build a thin, strong balloon. With the advice of a retired chemist, he used a small thin PVC material used as insulation for electrical wires to attempt to build that balloon, and it took hundreds of trials to come up with such a balloon.

On 12th February 1974 – Grüntzig used his new balloon on Mr Fritz Ott, a 67-year-old gentleman's leg, and like Mrs Shaw a decade earlier, it was a huge success, and a new technique was born.

Although Grüntzig used the term' new dilatation catheter' (neuer Dilatationskatheter), he still described his procedure as 'Dottern' in reference to the Seattle inventor Dr Charles Dotter.

The 49th American Heart Association meeting was held in Miami in November 1976. Gruintzig presented his work on coronaries dilation in animals in a poster session. Many of the audience were skeptical, but few were not, and one of them was Dr Richard Myler, a cardiologist from San Francisco who would become instrumental in developing PTCA [angioplasty].

On 22nd March 1977, the first patient had been denied surgery because of inoperable disease, but that attempt was unsuccessful because Gruintzig had to use the left arm to gain entry and was unable to cannulate the coronary arteries.

Gruintzig stated after that attempt: "If you start a method, you should start with an ideal case and not with end-stage disease."

Grüntzig wanted to try to dilate the stenotic coronary while the patient was on the operating table having his bypass surgery, but surgeons in Zurich refused to help him.

Dr Richard Myer from San Francisco, Dr. Grüntzig's new friend, convinced the surgeon Dr. Elias Hanna, who was born in Syria, to allow them to dilate the coronary stenosis while the patient was in the middle of the bypass surgery.

Dr Grüntzig did several of those dilatations with the help of Dr Myer in May of 1977.

Many of Grüntzig's colleagues in Zurich were not supportive. He was told by a very supportive surgeon Dr Senning, a pioneer himself, as he was the first to implant a pacemaker in a human.

Mister Grüntzig: Do it; if something happens, I will operate.

«Herr Grüntzig: Machen Sie es, falls etwas passiert, operiere ich!»

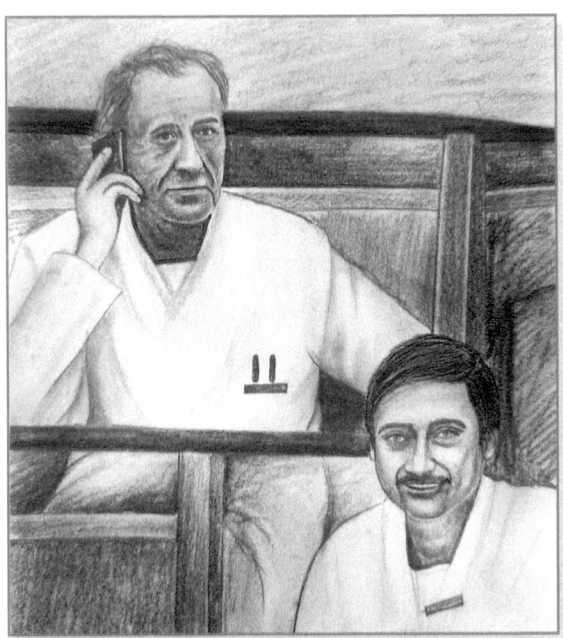

Dr Senning (left) and his protégé Dr Grüntzig

Grüntzig had to wait a while to find the ideal patient for his first angioplasty; on the 15th of September 1977, a day before the procedure, he went to the patient's room to explain to him the option of dilating his blocked artery.

Dolf Bachmann was a 38-year-old man, insurance salesman, and smoker with frequent and severe angina, requiring 20 nitroglycerin pills daily to control his pain and waiting for coronary artery bypass surgery (open heart surgery) for one blocked artery.

That afternoon, Grüntzig visited Mr. Bachmann in his hospital room, explained the procedure, and told him he would be the first human to receive such treatment.

Whatever the reason that made Mr. Bachmann accept, whether his youth, his fear of coronary bypass surgery, the fame he would gain, or Dr Grüntzig's detailed explanation and charm. The reason is not apparent.

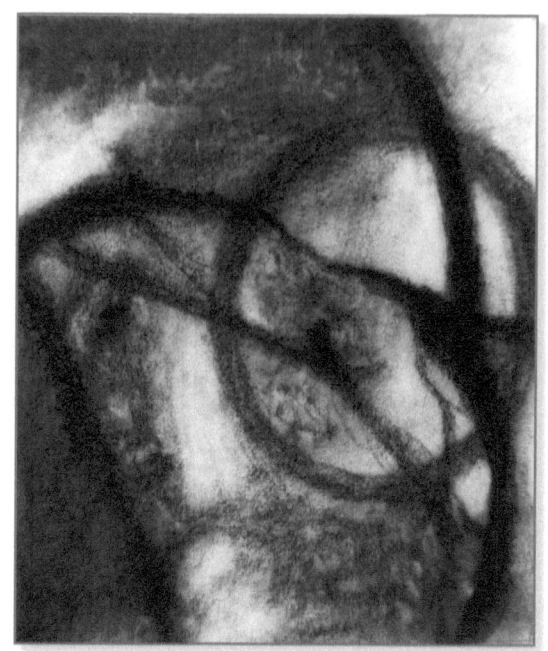

Dolf Bachmann's stenotic artery before PTCA in 1977

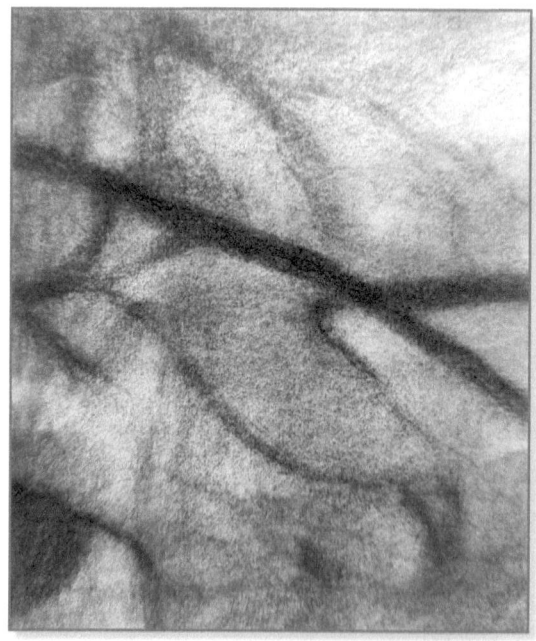

Dolf Bachmann's stenotic artery 2000

On 16th September, Mr. Bachmann became pain-free; later, he called a newspaper to spread the news.

Grüntzig was not happy and was able to convince Mr. Bachmann to cancel his scheduled interview with the reporter.

Grüntzig received very little support from his colleagues; he had to wait for two months before a patient was referred to him for a second coronary angioplasty.

However, he became famous abroad, and he held sessions for physicians from around the globe to watch him live, performing angioplasty.

He was limited to treating two patients weekly in Zurich, which made him think of transferring his skill to the US.

Many centers in the US wanted him to join them, among those Stanford, Harvard, and the Cleveland Clinic.

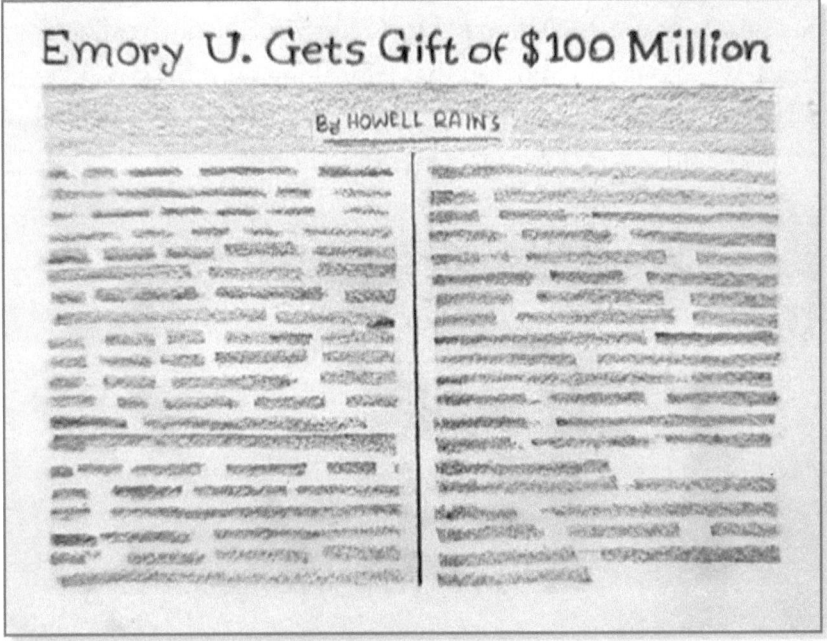

News Paper 11/08/1979

Emory University in Atlanta just received the highest research grant ever, 105 million dollars in the form of 3 million Coca-Cola shares. That was the deciding factor for Dr Grüntzig's choice of a new home.

As a result, on his transfer to Emory, he performed, in less than five years, more than 3000 thousand procedures 'without losing a single patient.'

He reflected on that later:

I was allowed to treat only two patients a week in Zurich. I could do two PTCA procedures a day when I came to Emory."

His favorite soft drink was Coca-Cola from that time, and he reasoned:

"When in Rome, do as the Romans do."

Fame and wealth were the Achilles tendon of Dr. Andreas Grüntzig. On 27th October 1985, while flying his airplane from his beach house to Atlanta, Dr. Grüntzig did not realize that death was his companion on that trip, along with his second wife Margaret-Ann Grüntzig, M.D., a radiology resident. She was 29 years old, and he was 46 years old.

CHAPTER 5

CHEMOTHERAPY

Bari is a small town in the south-eastern part of Italy; the British liberated it without a fight in September of 1943, and it became the main supply port for the Allied forces.

On 26th November 1943, the SS John Harvey, a US World War II Liberty ship, arrived at Bari carrying supplies and ammunition but was unable to unload its cargo on time because of congestion at the port.

On the night of December, the 2nd 1943, 105 German airplanes conducted an air raid on Bari; their targets were the Allied ships in its harbor.

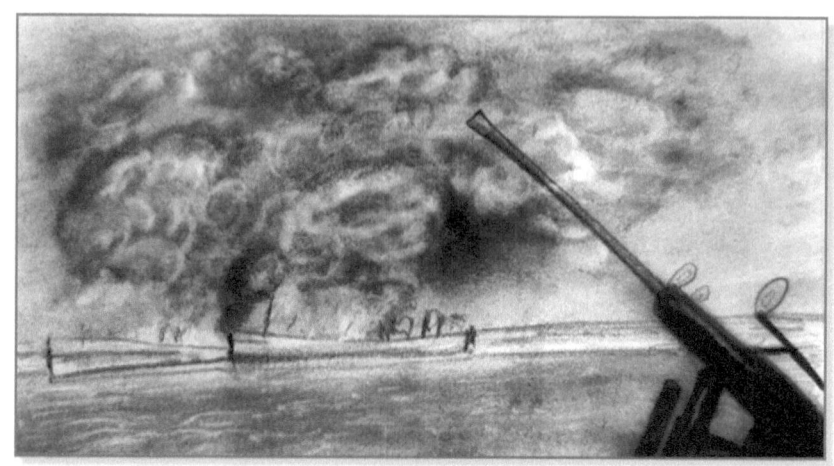

Air raid on Bari

Twenty-eight ships were sunk or destroyed, among them The SS John Harvey.

Very few people knew at the time that John Harvey was carrying a secret cargo consisting of mustard gas bombs.

Because of the prior intelligence report that the Germans had an advanced chemical weapon program and the widespread casualties with rapid speed among the victim of the German attack, the allied wanted to investigate whether it was a chemical attack by the Germans of some new type. Hence, the leadership on the ground in Bali requested assistance to investigate that possibility.

Five days after the attack, on 7th December at 5 pm, an American military plane touched down in Bari, carrying a young medical officer named Stewart Francis Alexander to lead the investigation.

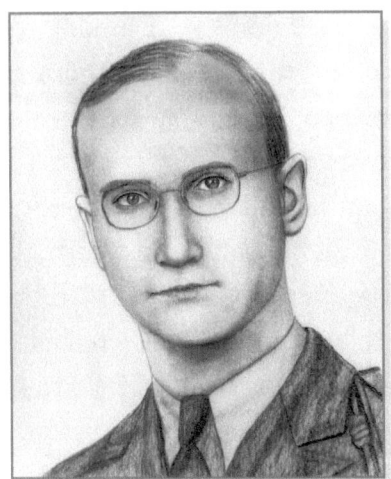
Dr Stewart Francis Alexander

His grandfather immigrated in late 1800 from Bratislava, the capital of today Slovakia; his father put himself through medical school by working long hours.

Dr Alexander volunteered in the Army medical corps like his father, who tried but failed to enlist in the Army in WWI. Dr Alexander was almost rejected because of poor vision after graduating from medical school.

During training, he discovered that the gas mask used by the Army did not fit well over his eyeglasses.

That prompted him to design a mask that soldiers who wore glasses could use. Naturally, that attracted the attention of the Chemical Warfare Service, and later he was transferred to that division and started his training in chemical warfare.

In Bari, he had the task of determining if a chemical weapon was used during that attack and what kind of gas, in case it was used.

Even though Hitler declined his general's request to use chemical weapons, the allied were not going to trust the German.

2000 Mustard Gas bombs were among the cargo of the SS John Harvey to be used in case the Germans used chemical weapons. Very few people knew of the nature of the shipment, and Dr alexander was not one of them.

Using his background training in chemical warfare, he noticed that many of the causalities lacked the sign of trauma to cause their demise; there were many skin burns, many of the victims had eyes injuries, and finally, a diver retrieved a part of a bomb that was tested positive for Mustard Gas.

His final report was rejected by Winston Churchill but was accepted by supreme commander, General Eisenhower.

Before writing his final report, he took many blood and tissue samples from the victims to study and analyze them. When his report was presented to his superior, it was immediately classified, meaning he could not discuss his finding without permission.

The German probably knew of the nature of the cargo, as Axis Sally, a failed American Broadway actress, turned German Radio announcer told her American GI audience, "I see you boys are getting gassed by your poison gas," her real name was Mildred Gillars.

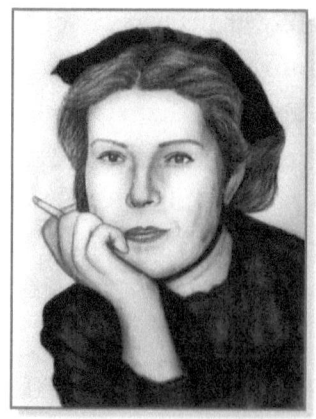

Axis Sally (Mildred Gillars)

Since WWI, it has been a known but forgotten fact that Mustard Gas caused a severe drop in white blood cell counts.

Part of Dr Alexander's responsibility in 1942, before the war, was to study the effect of a Mustard Gas derivative on humans, and he noticed the same drop in the white blood cell in rabbits given Mustard gas. However, he was forced to abandon his experiment because it did not benefit the war effort.

Dr Alexander did not give up and requested permission to seek outside counsel regarding his finding; it was granted in early 1942, several months before the Bari attack.

Dr Milton Charles Winternitz was his choice, the former dean of Yale medical school, who was dismissive of Dr Alexander's finding.

Dr Alexander did not know that Dr Winternitz had assigned two researchers from Yale to do the same experiment at about the same time. Dr Winternitz's action raises eyebrows and could not be explained.

For a few months, Goodman and Gilman, the two researchers from Yale, studied the effects of the Mustard Gas derivative on animals and confirmed its effect on the white blood cell in December 1942. They convinced Dr Linskog, a surgeon, to suggest this experimental treatment to a patient suffering from a rare kind of terminal cancer in the nose and throat.

Mr. DJ, a single Polish immigrant who failed radiation treatment, accepted the offer.

Despite the initial success, Mr. DJ died a couple of months later. He was the first human to receive a Mustard Gas derivative to treat his cancer.

Dr Cornelius P Rhoads, a peculiar person, Dr alexander's superior, played a major role in the advancement of chemotherapy.

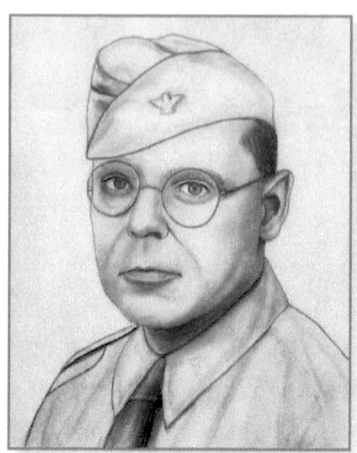

Dr Cornelius P Rhoads

A Graduate of Harvard in 1924, Dr Roads joined the Rockefeller Institute for Medical Research in 1928.

Before WWII, he enlisted in the US Army as a colonel and became the head of the chemical weapon program.

In 1931 and before enlisting in the Army, Dr Rhoads went to Puerto Rico to study anemia and tropical diseases as part of the Rockefeller Foundation research program.

One night, he emerged from a party to find his car vandalized; Dr Rhoads wrote a letter to his friend on the mainland:

"Puerto Ricans are beyond doubt the dirtiest, laziest, most degenerate and thievish race of men ever inhabiting this sphere. The island needs not public health work but a tidal wave or something to exterminate the population. I have done my best to further the extermination process by killing off eight and transplanting cancer into several more."

He never mailed that letter, but a lab technician discovered it, and a copy was sent to the newspapers and even to the Vatican.

Dr Rhoads left the island for New York, not willing to face the uproar among the native Puerto Ricans.

He was embraced and protected by the Rockefeller Foundation, and even the foundation's spin doctor, Ivy Lee, was hired to handle the bad publicity in New York that letter caused.

Mr. Lee influenced both the Times and New York Times articles to present the letter as a 'joke' and never intended to be mailed.

An investigation was conducted, and again under the Rockefeller influence, it was concluded in 2 weeks, and that brief investigation found no evidence of any crime committed. Dr Cornelius Rhoads went back to work for the Rockefeller Foundation. This episode deepened the colonial sentiment among the natives.

Dr Alexander filed his report regarding the Bali incident with his superior, Dr Cornelius Rhoads. As the head of the Chemical Warfare Service, he was in contact with the Yale group, who treated the first patient with Mustard Gas derivative with little success.

The Yale group tried treating five additional cancer patients with no success, and after that, each team member went his own way.

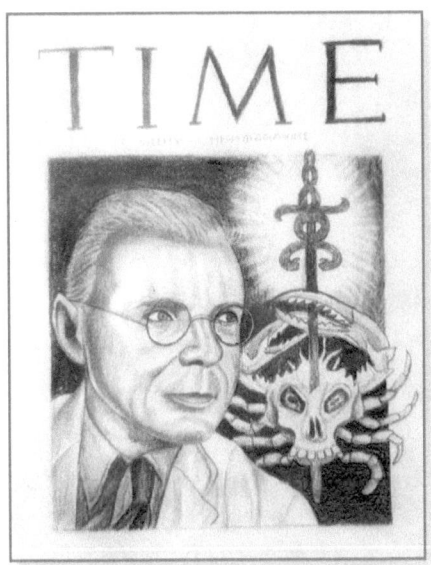

After the war, Dr Cornelius Rhoads convinced two executives from General Motors to donate 4 million dollars for cancer research. This was achieved using the Yale experience data and the Bari report, which documented the melting away of the lymphocyte (one kind of white blood cell) in the blood and bone marrow of the victims exposed to the mustard gas.

The Sloan Kettering Institute for Cancer Research became the mecca for many researchers and physicians to collaborate in the fight against cancer.

The fight against cancer was never without sets back, as demonstrated by the case of the Sloan Kettering Institute's most notorious patient, Babe Ruth. After failing all other treatments in 1948, the patient received chemotherapy for a rare Nasopharyngeal cancer (throat and nose). However, after an initial short success period, Babe Ruth's cancer relapsed, and he died shortly after.

On the other hand, a collaboration between Sloan Kettering Institute, initiated by Dr Rhoads, with two researchers, Gertrude Elion and George Hitchings, from the pharmaceutical firm Burroughs, Welcome & Co produced a new chemotherapy called 6MP, which was approved at the end of 1953.

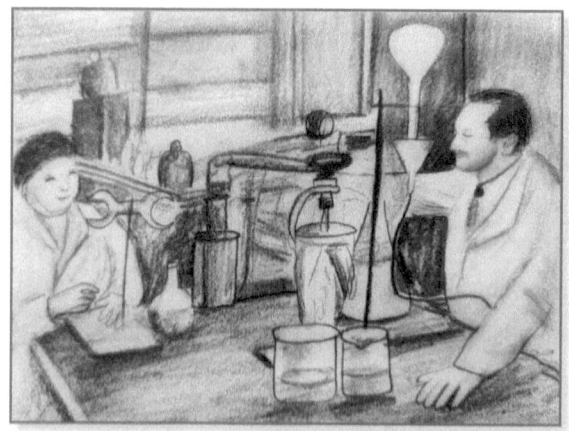

Gertrude Elion and George Hitchings

In 1954, Debbie Brown was a nine-year-old girl diagnosed with leukemia and had to be homeschooled because of her illness.

She was treated by a member of the Sloan Kettering Institute with a combination of 6 MP and another newly discovered chemotherapy called methotrexate.

Her response was remarkable and long-lasting; she graduated from high school, married, had a child, and became a teacher.

CHAPTER 6

CONTRACEPTIVE

It took our ancestors, perhaps millions of years, to recognize that pregnancy is directly related to intercourse because many sexual activities did not end with a pregnancy.

The one that ends up with pregnancy, its result would not be recognized immediately, but several weeks later. A long time would pass between the intercourse and the pregnancy, so the cause-effect relationship is often blurry and unclear.

The first possible archaeological proof of this relationship was found in Çatalhöyük, a small gathering of 8000 people who lived 9000 years ago in present-day Turkey. A plaque was found of a mother and child on one side and two figures embracing each other, on the other side of the plaque, suggesting the embracing produced the child.

Later, it became clear, and the father's role with his duties and responsibilities were spelled out in the Hammurabi code in Babylon 1755-1750 BC.

There was no need for contraceptives initially due to high infant mortality and multiple deliveries to compensate for the lost one.

Also, a prolonged lactation period was practiced at the time, as mothers were nursing their children for 2-3 years, which would make pregnancy less likely, because of the suppression of ovulation.

The need for contraceptives varies among societies, cultures, religions, and eras.

One would imagine that conception outside of marriage in ancient times was one of the most important reasons for the demand because women needed contraceptives to avoid shame and violence.

Perhaps economic reasons followed in urbanized societies and became essential after women started working out of their homes, but the demand for contraceptives was still minimal.

In the 19 century, contraceptive methods were ineffective, sometimes intrusive and occasionally extremely dangerous, which is why they were very unpopular.

Mechanical means were the most common birth control methods, and the rhythm methods were largely ineffective because the calculations were based on observations of animals which was incorrect.

The absentee period was thought erroneously to be around menstruation, the least fertile period in the women's productive cycle.

Margaret Sanger 1879–1966 played a pivotal role in the birth control Pill's discovery. Her mother, Anne Higgins, died of tuberculosis at age 50 after 18 pregnancies, so Margaret decided to be a nurse and advocate for women's causes.

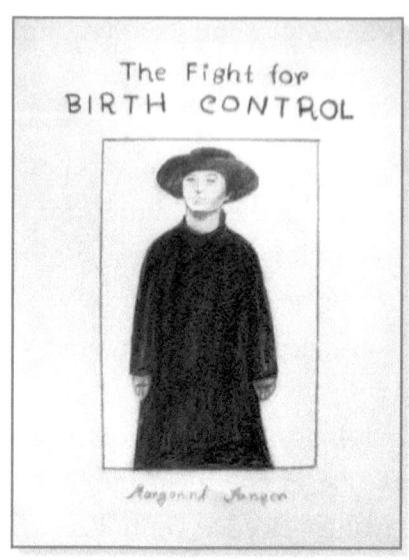

Margaret Sanger

In 1912, she settled with her family in New York City and worked as a nurse in poverty-stricken areas, the Lower East Side of New York City. This was where she was exposed to poverty and sickness, partially due to multiple pregnancies, so she became convinced of the need for inexpensive and effective birth control.

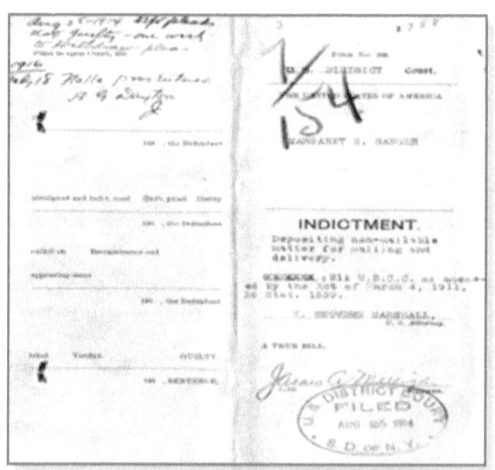

Indictment

She published a newspaper, 'The Woman Rebel,' advocating women's rights and discussing matters relating to women, especially women from the working class, that included birth control advice.

The post office issued a warrant for her arrest for publishing advice on birth control under the infamous law, The Comstock Act of 1873. That law prohibits sending "obscene, lewd or lascivious," "immoral," or "indecent" publications through the mail.

She jumped bail and went to Europe; in 1915, she asked her husband for divorce while she was still in Europe; however, her husband was arrested and served 30 days jail sentence under the same law, which convinced Margaret to return home.

In 1916, Margaret opened the first birth control clinic in Brooklyn, NY, which was raided ten days later by the post office police.

A large crowd of her supporter marched outside the courtroom; while she admitted in court,ownership of the banned birth control pamphlets, the three judges' panels, not wanting to make her a martyr, decided to release Margret if she agreed not to violate the law again.

Margaret answered, "I cannot promise to obey a law I do not respect," so the chief judge gave her a choice of a fine or jail sentence. She chose to spend 30 days in jail, refused to be fingerprinted, and refused her physical examination. She considered herself a political prisoner.

After seven years of separation from her husband, Margaret married a wealthy widower named James Noah Slee, 20 years older than her. That gave her significant financial support and increased her ability to be introduced to influential individuals.

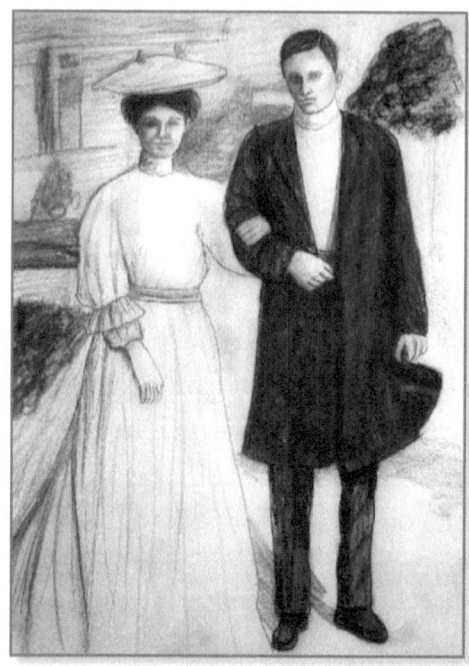

Katharine Dexter McCormick (1875-1967)

Another woman who played a significant part in the Pill development was Katherine Dexter (1875 – 1967); she was born in Michigan to a wealthy family. She graduated from MIT in 1904 with a Bachelor of Science in Biology to be the second women graduate from this famous institution.

An independent and outspoken woman, Katharine forced MIT to change its policy that forced female students to wear feathered hats on the ground that it could be a fire hazard.

Katharine married Stanley McCormick, of Chicago, a Princeton-educated man and heir to a vast fortune in 1904, who was diagnosed with schizophrenia just years after their wedding.

Stanley's illness had a sexual expression and violent attitude against women, so she was not allowed to be in close contact with him for over twenty years.

She kept in contact through letters and phone calls, and she occasionally had to use a pair of binoculars to see him.

Throughout her husband's illness and isolation, she remained married to him until he died in 1947.

She was in constant conflict with his sibling because she believed his illness might be due to hormonal imbalance, and his treatment needed to be changed.

She devoted her life to women's issues; initially, it was the women's suffrage movement. She became a National American Woman Suffrage Association member and later the association's vice president in 1914.

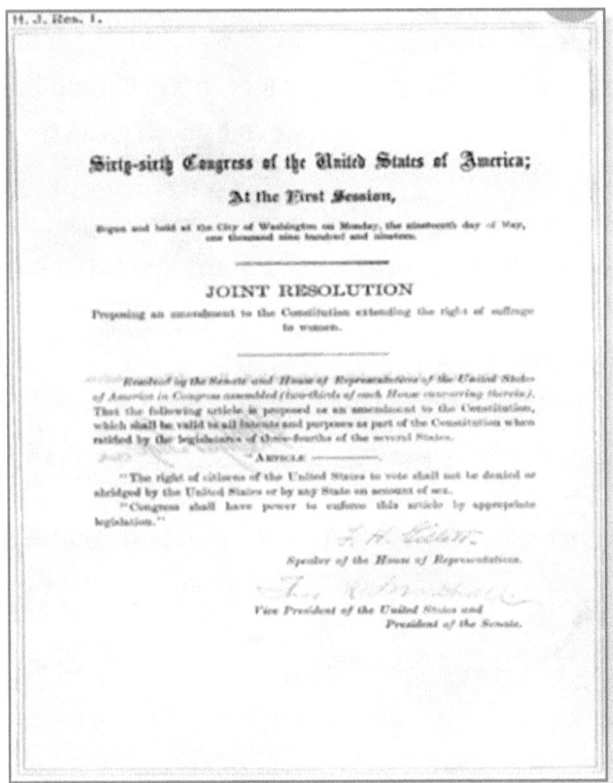

The nineteenth amendment

After ratification of the nineteenth amendment, guaranteeing the women's right to vote, she turns her attention and effort to birth control.

Schizophrenia at the time was thought to be hereditary; some historians Connect Katherine McCormick's interest in birth control with her husband's diagnosis, she did not want to have children.

Other historians connected her interest in birth control with her experience at MIT because, despite her success in passing the entrance exam at MIT, she was asked to take additional courses; this made her think that she was singled out because she was a woman.

In 1922, Kathryn McCormick was part of a smuggling scheme to bring the illegal diaphragm to the United States from Europe. She stuffed them into her coats and garments to escape the custom agent.

Because of her significant interest in the relationship between endocrine disorder and schizophrenia, believing that her husband's illness was endocrine in origin, and because of her contentious relationship with her in-law, she needed to avoid financing a controversial cause. She directed some of her donations to that cause and established the Neuroendocrine Research Foundation at Harvard Medical School in 1927.

After her husband death in 1947. She had complete control of her financial fortune; it took her two more years to settle her inheritance taxes problem.

Kathryn McCormick wrote in 1948 to Margret Sanger, the champion of birth control, offering help and support.

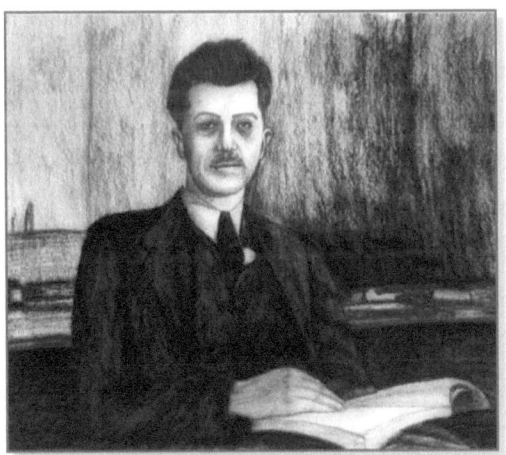

Gregory Pincus (1903-1967)

Gregory Pincus was born in 1903 to a family of Russian-Jewish immigrants; he spent his college year at Cornell University supporting himself by washing dishes.

He moved on to Harvard and was granted a postgraduate fellowship soon after he got involved in animal experiments related to fertilization.

At the age of 31, he attracted attention because he fertilized a rabbit's egg in a test tube and transplanted that egg to a host, radical research at that time, the New York time called him "Dr Frankenstein".

His time at Harvard came to an end because of that bad publicity; he could not find any job at any other institution.

His classmate rescued him from Harvard, and he was able to find a job at Clark University in Massachusetts; he kept working with hormones.

In 1944 Pincus and his classmate established the Worcester Foundation for Experimental Biology, A private lab lacking the financial resources; he worked as the lab's janitor to support himself.

Gregory Pincus was the scientist, and his partner Hudson Hoagland became the fundraiser; they became a successful couple raising enough money to conduct more research on the hormone's effect on rabbits' reproductive system and neurobehavior biology. One of those contributors was Catharine McCormick, who was influenced by her schizophrenic husband's condition.

In 1951, Margaret Sanger met Gregory Pincus at a dinner party in New York City; knowing his research interest was in hormones, she asked if he could help discover the magic pill. To her surprise, the answer was affirmative, but it will require a significant amount of funding.

Margaret Sanger knew the perfect person to call; it was Katharine McCormick, her wealthy women friend who had called Margaret a year earlier offering help.

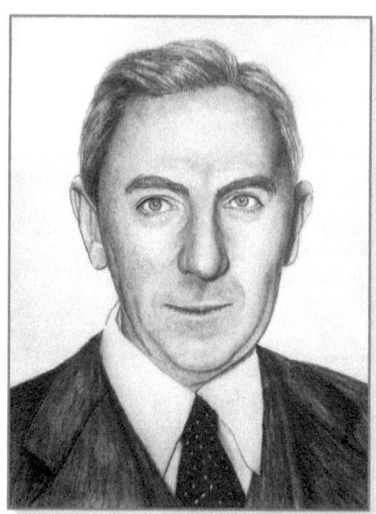

Dr John Rock

Gregory Pincus recognized from the beginning that he needed a physician and preferably a gynecologist on his team for the project to be successful.

Dr John Rock, a Harvard graduate, was his choice for the job. He was a respected gynecologist by his peers. He was also admired by his patient, a devoted Catholic who worked on a controversial project and became the spokesperson who promoted birth control pills.

Gregory Pincus was aware of the work done in 1919 by Ludwig Haberlandt (1885 - 1932), an Austrian physiologist, who induced a state of temporary sterilization in an animal after transforming follicular cells (cells from the ovaries) from a pregnant animal to the first one.

Ludwig Haberlandt tried to convince his colleague and drug companies to produce a hormonal contracept drug, to no avail and ended up committing suicide.

On the negative side, Gregory Pincus knew of the monumental objections to developing birth control pills. Thirty States banned birth control products' sale or even advertisement. The Catholic Church's position at that time was obvious; producing or using birth control products is sinful.

From a market perspective, business executives thought that it would be hard to develop a large market for birth control pills because a healthy woman would resent taking a pill daily not to prevent or treat any diseases.

The cost of natural progesterone therapy made it unaffordable for the average person as the gram cost over $80. On top of that the drug administration was impractical as it had to be injected.

In 1951, simultaneously, Carl Djerassi of syntax in Mexico, and Frank Colton of G. D. Searle in Chicago, were successful in producing synthesized progesterone at a fraction of the price, which could be given orally, and they became the progesterone supplier to Gregory Pincus and his team.

A small trial conducted In Massachusetts was labeled intentionally, as a fertility trial by Pincus and Rock, to avoid violating any existing laws prohibiting counterpetition.

The trial results were not very promising, but the good news was that no one died or got seriously ill, although few women became pregnant.

Also, many women falsely thought they were pregnant because of their menstrual period interruption and because they had side effects similar to the symptoms of pregnancy.

A simple solution was found, which is to restore menstruation and keep prohibiting ovulation; so, women were told to skip the pill five days a month.

The next step is a large trial to obtain FDA approval for the pill; that trial could not be conducted in most states because of existing laws.

Puerto Rico was chosen to be the place for this large trial even though most of the population was Catholic, because the only choice before the contraceptive pill was sterilization, which was popular among the poor population. It was simply referred to as "la operacion."

There were many reasons for choosing Puerto Rico; the most important one was that the existing law did not prohibit contraception practices, plus the existence of a large poor population in a crowded area, as volunteers!

Although critics raised many questions about using the poor, uneducated population as Guinea pigs, some went further by labeling the trial as a form of colonialism and the exploitation of poor women. Using as a proof, what Pincus wrote in The Washington Post on Aug 2, 1959:

"The control of the population explosion now upon us by the limitations of births is particularly demanding in countries where the birth-rate pressure curtails already limited economic development."

The study was criticized for substandard practices, as side effects were dismissed and thought to be due to psychosomatic reasons by the investigators. More importantly, three women's deaths during the trial were not investigated, and autopsies were not done to see if their deaths were related to the pill. Keeping the bad news in the closet.

Finally, a few critics attacked one of the study supporters and contributors, Clarence Gamble, for being a member of the "Human Betterment League of North Carolina", a eugenics group.

Despite all the justifiable reasons critics gave, the trial continued and Enovid (the pill) was approved officially as a contraceptive on May 11, 1960, by FDA.

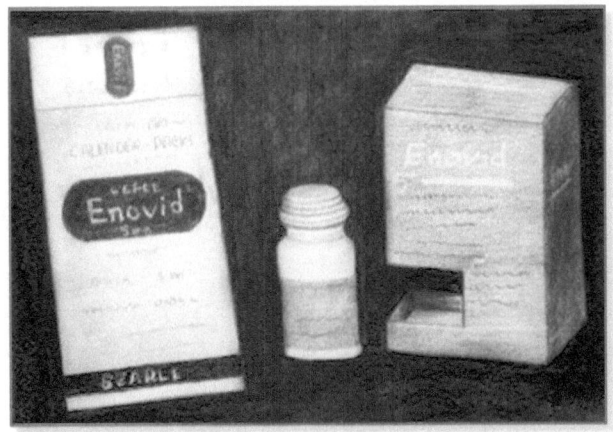

Enovid

CHAPTER 7

CORTISONE

In 1855 Thomas Addison described 11 patients with a new disease, what is now known as Addison disease; but focusing on the anemia part of the syndrome created some speculation among historians about the accuracy of his discovery, but that speculation was proven wrong later on.

The new disease was due to adrenal gland insufficiency, and his autopsy findings were remarkable, as they described the destruction of the adrenal glands in those patients.

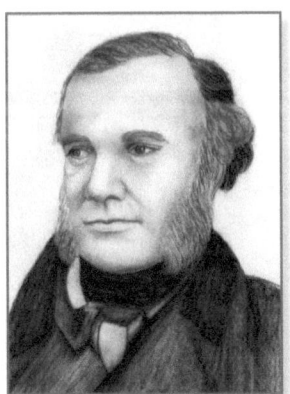

Thomas Addison

In 1856, Charles-Edouard Brown-Séquard was born in Mauritius to a French mother and an American father. His father was a sailor who died in the sea before his son was born. Brown-Séquard was a British citizen because Mauritius was a British colony in the Indian Ocean.

He became a physiologist and the first to declare that adrenal glands were "organs essential for life". Since the animals died shortly after he removed their adrenal glands, and that death was not due to bleeding or infection.

He further demonstrated that the animal survived when transfused with blood from a normal animal.

In a lecture at the University of Paris later (1869), he suggested that the 'glands have internal secretions and furnish to the blood useful if not essential principles.'

The Brown-Séquard view was not accepted because the medical community thought, at that time, that the adrenal glands were like the appendix, inconsequential.

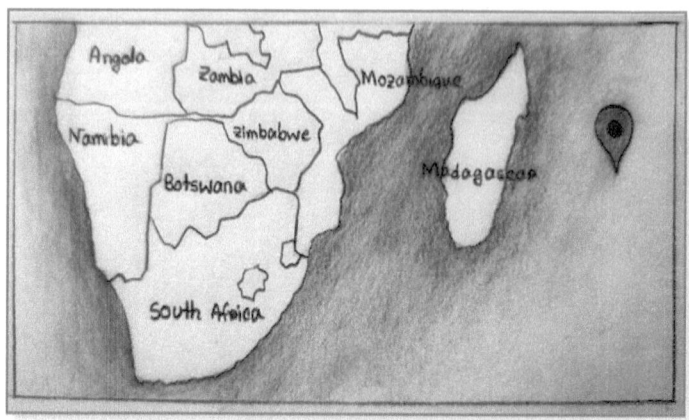

Mauritius

Sir William Osler (1849 –1919) was a Canadian physician, a pioneer in medical education and training; he was the first to bring medical students from the classroom to the bedside and one of four physicians who founded John Hopkins Hospital.

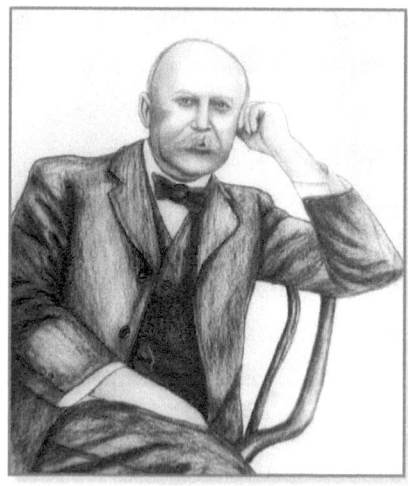

Sir William Osler

William Osler was the first to administer Adrenal extract to a patient with Addison's disease in 1896.

First, he had to produce the suprarenal extract from 36 pigs.

He described his patient, upon discharge after the treatment, "got much better and went back to work."

During the 1940s, Nazi troops were supplied with methamphetamine, a stimulus called "Pervitin," According to British War Office, from April to June 1940, about 35 million Pervitin tablets were sent to 3 million German soldiers, seamen and pilots.

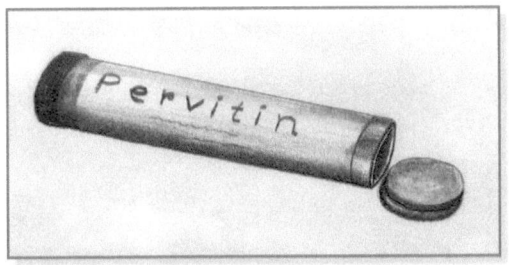

On the other hand, the American and British soldiers were supplied with amphetamine, another stimulus; in the North African campaign in 1942, over half a million Benzedrine tablets "Speed" were distributed on the orders of Gen. Dwight D. Eisenhower.

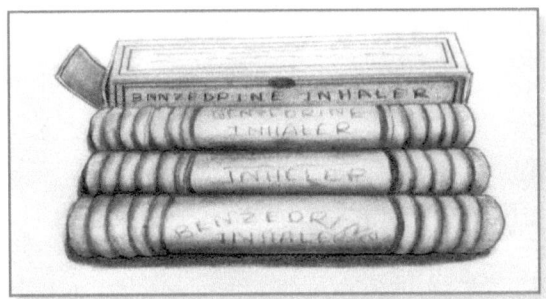

In 1941, an Intelligence source thought the Germans were giving their pilots a substance extracted from the adrenal gland of cattle imported from Argentina. That substance was supposed to keep the pilots and the personnel in airplanes and submarines longer.

In response, the American and British governments poured resources into the research of the adrenal gland to try to isolate the effective substances.

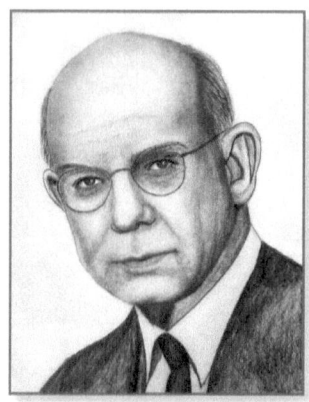

Edward Calvin Kendall (1886 – 1972)

Edward Kendall, a chemist at the Mayo Clinic, was receiving shipments of adrenal tissues from Chicago slaughterhouses to try to isolate substances with clinical benefit.

In 1942, a chemist from Merck and Company, Lewis Sarett, worked for three months in Kendall's laboratory.

At the end of that effort, they produced 28 compounds, four of which were thought to be the most promising: A, B, E, and F.

The yields of these attempts were low, with only 85 to 500 mg of the effective compounds isolated from 50 kg of adrenal glands.

Therefore, it was initially agreed that these compounds' use should be limited to studies with small animals, and none should be used in clinical medicine.

Since those substances could restore post-adrenalectomy animals' ability to resist toxins, they were tried sporadically in humans suffering from trauma and a certain type of infection, but the results were not very promising.

Finally, in May of 1948, Merck and Co Inc produced a few grams of compound E without any idea of what clinical application should be investigated.

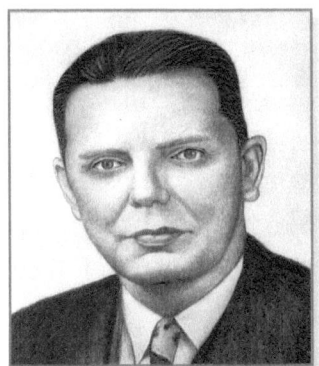

Philip Showalter Hench, 1896–1965

On 1st April 1929, Dr Hench described a case of a 65-year-old physician who had rheumatoid arthritis, The patient's symptoms improved after he became jaundiced, and his improvement lasted for several months past the jaundice episode.

In 1933, Hench reported a similar phenomenon in seven patients; finally, his collection grew to 31 patients in 1938. Some patients had jaundice, some were pregnant, some suffered from infection, and others had undergone recent surgery.

Attempts to reproduce his finding by the administration of bile or by transfusing jaundiced blood failed. This made him think that it was not the bile which produced the improvement but some other internal "substance X", which was internally produced due to jaundice, and that was the reason for the improvement.

Then, on 21st September 1948, the first intramuscular injection of compound E was administered to a woman who had severe rheumatoid arthritis and had been hospitalized for over a month because she refused to go home in a wheelchair. That took place at the Mayo Clinic.

She had a remarkable improvement, and it was said that: 'she walked out of the hospital in a gay mood and went on a shopping trip.'

Similar successes were achieved on 30 more patients over the next seven months. One of those patients took several baths on the same day because she was denied this pleasure for so long.

Initially, Hench tried to keep the story and the success of cortisone in a small circuit until a complete understanding of the benefits and the complications were studied. Still, a reporter from the New York Times was tipped off, and he published stories and pictures about cortisone that forced Hench to announce the discovery in May 1949.

In 1950, the Nobel Prize in Physiology or Medicine was awarded to Philip Showalter Hench, his colleague Edward Calvin Kendall, and the Polish-Swiss chemist Tadeus Reichstein, who had discovered cortisone independently about the same time.

Dr Hench shared the financial reward from the Nobel Prize with his colleagues. Sister Pantaleon, the nursing supervisor, who refused to accept the money because she vowed to poverty, so Dr Hench created a study grant, so sister Pantaleon could go to Europe and meet the Pope.

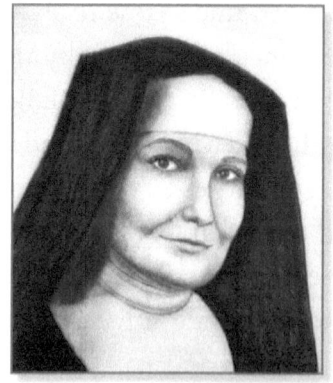

Sister Pantaleon

CHAPTER 8

COUMADIN / WARFARIN

In the early 1920s, farmers were struggling financially, and their cattle were struck with a mysterious disease, killing a large number with extensive internal and external bleeding.

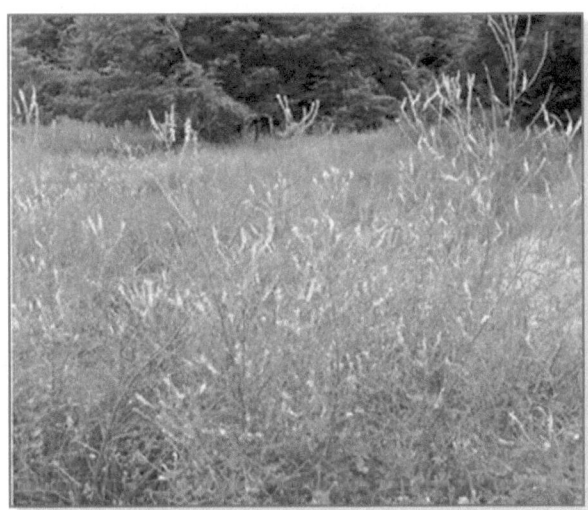

Sweet Clover

Frank Schofield, an English veterinarian who emigrated to Canada, discovered that the outbreak was due to the animals eating moldy sweet clover hay. Since he found out that all affected cattle had eaten the same moldy hay, and when he fed rabbits the same hay, the rabbits became inflicted by the same disease.

Without knowing the exact cause of the disease, he recommended feeding the animals other kinds of hay.

In the winter of 1933, a farmer from Wisconsin named Ed Carlson lost five of his cows to the same disease, and his most valuable bull started bleeding from his nose.

Mr. Carlson drove 190 miles with a dead cow and a can full of blood that did not clot with several pounds of spoiled sweet clover and went to the University of Wisconsin's Agricultural Department for help. This is because he could not afford different hay in the midst of the great depression.

Karl Paul Link was a head researcher at the University of Wisconsin Agricultural Department; he changed the department's research subject to investigate that mysterious disease.

One of Link's associates isolated the hemorrhagic agent and found that the hemorrhagic agent was formed when an enzyme in the fungus, which caused the hay to mold, combined several molecules, and that new agent caused the cattle to bleed; the mystery was solved.

Link became sick in 1945 and could not work for several months. During that time, he read many books, including "The History of rodent control from Ancient to Modern Times".

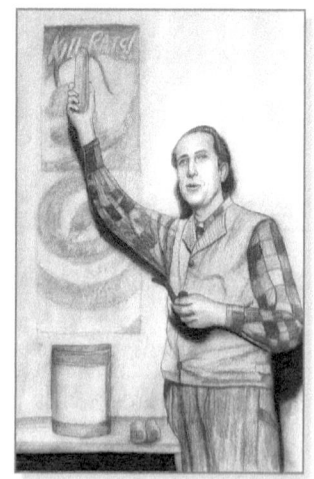

Karl Paul Link

This book led him to the idea of using that hemorrhagic agent as rat Poison, it had no taste and no odor, and it does not kill the rat immediately since the rats are not dumb, and they would not touch the poison if they realized it was killing their peer.

Out of the more than 100 variations of that agent, Link tested them using variable animals to find the most effective, and its compound 42.

He named The Wisconsin Alumni Research Foundation, which had supported the research, the holder of the patent, also the compound was called Warfarin, the initials of the foundation.

Link tried to convince medical researchers to investigate any role of Warfarin in the medical field. Still, his attempts were rejected because they all thought using and marketing a drug used as rat poison was a crazy idea.

On April 4, 1951, a 22-year-old US Navy inductee attempted suicide in Philadelphia, and was admitted with abdominal and back pain, and perfused nosebleed.

After he became more alert, he told his doctors that he was attempting suicide. He also revealed to the doctor that he took a small amount of the rat poison without any effects, so he kept taking it four days in a row and finally became ill on the fifth day.

His successful treatment by transfusion and vitamin K encouraged many researchers to begin treatment trials with warfarin, which was approved by the FDA in 1954.

Another event that helped to transform Warfarin from a rat poison to a trusted medication was President Eisenhower's heart attack, which he suffered in September 1955; the president was treated with warfarin and mistakenly thought, at the time, that it was a successful treatment.

Over the decade, there have been speculations that the Soviet dictator Joseph Satin was poisoned with warfarin. As late as 2003, those speculations were circulating in the popular media, like the New York times.

In all those accounts, they claimed that Stalin was poisoned the night before he collapsed.

Despite all the circumstantial evidence presented to raise those speculations, the fact is that warfarin, as a poison, does not cause bleeding in a short time but requires several days.

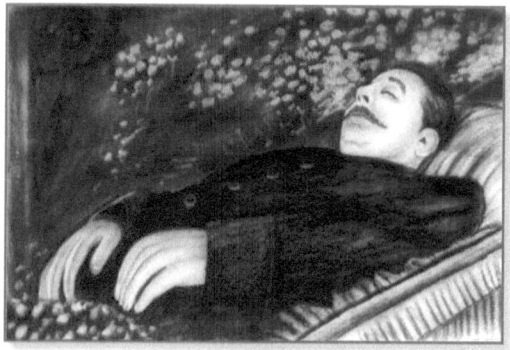

Joseph Stalin

CHAPTER

DIABETES

At the dawn of the 20th century, diabetes was a rare disease. Diabetes has increased since, becoming one of humanity's most common and costly diseases.

Only 172 patients with diabetes were admitted to Massachusetts General Hospital out of 47,899 total admissions between the years 1824 and 1898.

The accurate prevalence of diabetes was not well known until the 1950s because the diagnosis was unavailable and not consistently accurate.

It was not until 1922 that diabetes made the ten most common cause of death in the United States disappear from the list again till 1932, and since then, it has become the number 7 on that list.

In recent times, there have been nearly 26 million patients with diabetes in the United States; that is 8.3% of the population at the cost of nearly 245 billion dollars a year. Two-thirds of that is a direct cost, and one-third is indirect cost like disability and work loss, according to American Diabetic Association.

In the ancient Egyptian Ebbers papyrus, dated back to 1500 BC, some historians believe there is a description of the symptoms of diabetes, excessive thirst, and copious urination.

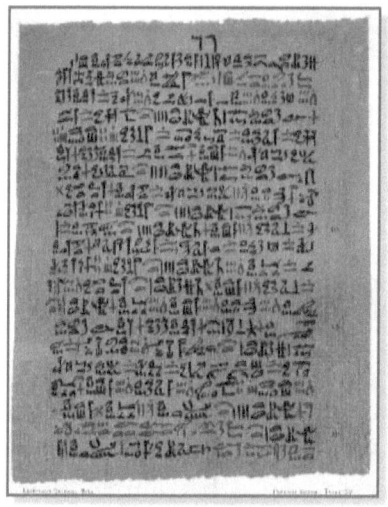

Ebbers papyrus

Sushruta, an Indian physician (7th or 6th century BCE), described patients with Diabetes and used the term Madhumeha (honey-like urine) because their urine not only tasted sweet but also attracted ants.

Aretaeus of Cappadocian lived in Rome probably in the 2nd century AD and Introduced the term 'diabetes'. Its origin is the Greek verb διαβαινω (diabaino) which means "pass-through" because diabetic patients drink a lot of water and frequently urinate as if the water runs through them.

In the 11th century AD, The Islamic physician Avicenna (980-1037), in his book El-Kanun, described some diabetes complications like gangrene and sexual dysfunction.

The English physician Thomas Willis lived in the 17th century, added the word 'Mellitus' to the name, a Latin word for sweet, due to the sweet taste of the urine in people with diabetes, unaware of Sucheta's observation a century earlier.

In 1772, Peter Dickerson, a 33-year-old man, was admitted to the hospital because he passed one pint of urine every hour; his treating physician was Matthew Dobson.

Dr Dickerson described his patient's urine as sweet; more importantly, his blood tasted sweet as well.

Dobson published his account in the Medical Observations and Inquiries journal in 1776. It was the journal of a medical society in London, a select group of physicians who met on alternate Monday evenings at the MITRE Tavern on Fleet Street.

He boiled the urine of Peter Dickerson and confirmed that the residue had the taste of sugar.

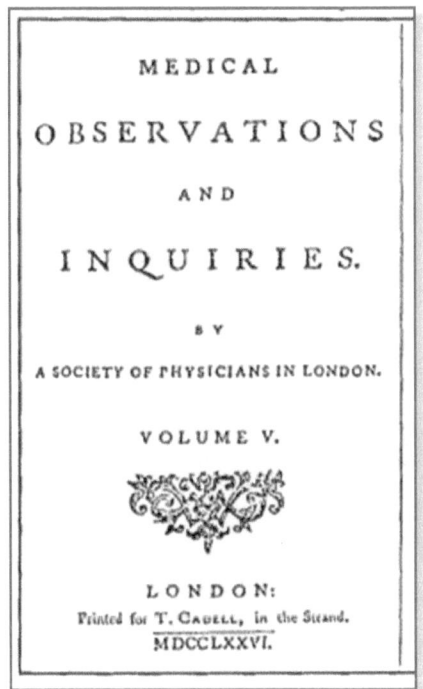

The process of detecting sugar in the urine was developed in 1841, but it was not until 1913 that the quantitative measurement of blood sugar was invented.

In the 19th century, many scientists thought that the pancreas must have a role in diabetes development, as they found pancreatic atrophy in postmortem examination of diabetic patients.

Oskar Minkowski (1858-1931) and Joseph Von Mering (1849-1908) removed the pancreas of a dog, that made the dog diabetic, and this opened the door for further evaluation of the relationship between the pancreas and diabetes.

The experiment was repeated on three dogs; all had sugar in their urine.

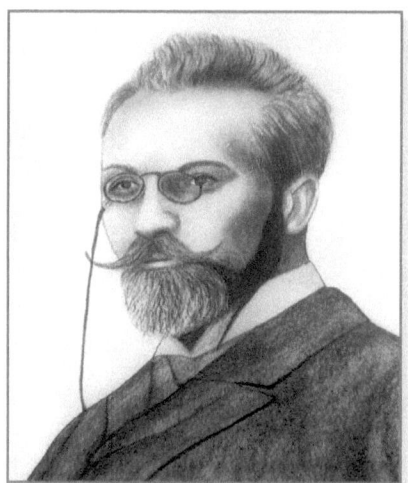

Oskar Minkowski

Minkowski implanted a small portion of the pancreas in one of those dogs and noticed that the blood sugar returned to normal until the piece of the pancreas was removed.

Frederick Banting, the 1923 Noble Prize winner, wrote about his co-Noble prize winner, John Macleod.

"Macleod, on the other hand, was never to be trusted. He

was the most selfish man I have ever known. He sought every possible opportunity to advance himself. If you told Macleod anything in the morning, it was in print or a lecture in his name by evening. He was unscrupulous and would steal an idea or credit for work from any possible source."

Banting thought that Macleod did not deserve any recognition, as his role in insulin discovery was more a supportive role than a discoverer.

Frederick Banting was an orthopedic physician who had just returned from the horror of the First World War and was approached in 1921 by the director of the physiology lab at the University of Toronto, John MacLeod. He presented a novel idea on how to extract insulin from the pancreatic extract of an animal.

Before that, many attempts have been unsuccessful in extracting pure insulin from the animal's pancreas.

The pancreas has two different functions. On the one hand, it secretes insulin; on the other hand, it secretes enzymes that break down protein. And since insulin is protein, those enzymes make extracting insulin almost impossible.

Macleod teamed Banting with Charles Best, a final-year honors student, and provided Banting with the lab space, lab animals, and financial support.

Finally, he infused the team with a biochemist named James Collip.

Insulin was isolated by ligating the pancreatic duct, which led to pancreatic atrophy, without affecting the isles cell responsible for insulin secretions.

To their happy surprise, after the insulin injection in a dog, its pancreas was removed, and within hours, the blood sugar started dropping. The experiment was conducted several times on other dogs and achieved similar results.

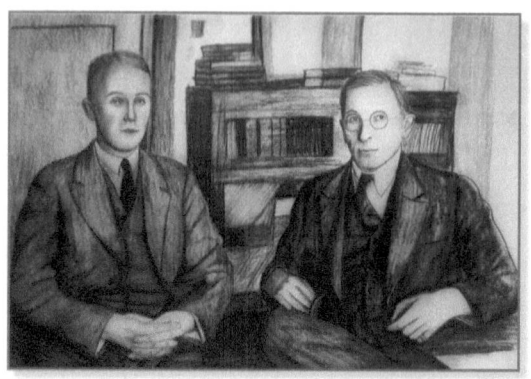

Charles Best and Frederick Banting

Leonard Thompson, a 14-year-old boy, was being treated for diabetes in Toronto Hospital, and on the 11th of January 1922, the newly discovered insulin was administered to Leonard, who was markedly sick. Unfortunately, the first injection in the buttock was unsuccessful and was complicated by infection at the injection site.

Leonard received a second injection 12 days later, and to everybody's surprise, he felt better, and his blood sugar dropped from 520 to 120 in 24 hours; he lived for another 13 years.

Another patient was Elizabeth Hughes Gossett (1907-1981), the daughter of a United States politician. She was diagnosed with diabetes at age 11 and started treatment with insulin in August 1922; she responded well to the treatment, survived, and graduated from college. She married, had three children, and died suddenly of a heart attack at age 74.

The Nobel Prize committee awarded the noble prize in 1923 to only two of the four people who worked on inventing insulin, John Macleod and Frederick Banting.

Frederick Banting was furious and believed that Charles Best deserved the prize more than John MacLeod, so Frederick shared his cash prize with Charles Best, which made MacLeod also share his award with Collip.

CHAPTER 10

HYPERTENSION

Ancient civilizations had little knowledge of hypertension and its effect on human health and longevity.

In 1733 the English clergyman, Stephen Hales, was the first to measure the blood pressure of a mare by inserting a Brass pipe into one of the mare's arteries and connecting that pipe with a 9 feet glass tube, watching the blood rises to over 8 feet.

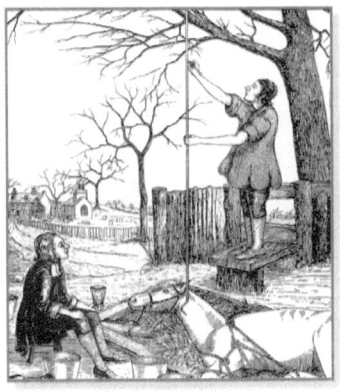

Stephen Hales

Not until 1896 did the Italian Scipione Riva-Rocci Invent a modern and near-accurate way to measure blood pressure non-invasively, without surgery.

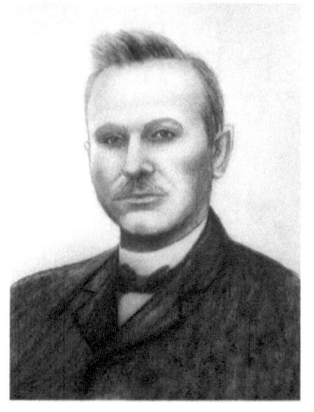 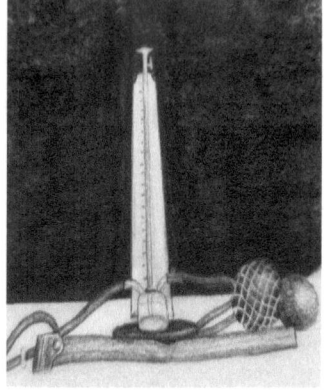

Scipione Riva-Rocci   *Scipione's blood pressure machine*

He improved the earlier version of the blood pressure machine called the sphygmomanometer by applying a general principle.

That principle states that the pressure inside the artery equals the pressure needed to occlude the artery and prevent the blood flow distally.

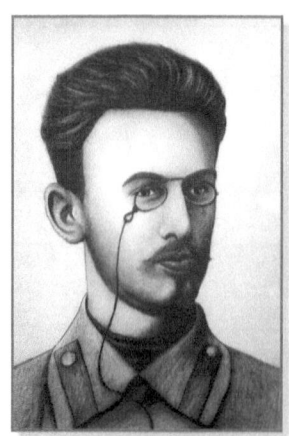

Nikolai Korotkoff

In 1905, Nikolai Korotkoff published a brief and modest paper of 207 words describing a simple measurement method for blood pressure systolic "upper number "and diastolic "lower number ".

He contributed by adding the use of a stethoscope to determine when the blood stopped flowing, which indicates systolic hypertension, and when it resumed regular flowing, which measures diastolic pressure.

Nikolai Korotkoff's invention withstood the test of time, as we still use it today.

The life insurance community recognized the effect of hypertension on mortality long before the medical community did.

A few decades later, In the first edition of the "gold standard" pharmacologic textbook, only ten references to hypertension or its therapy were included in a volume of more than 1300 pages.

Up to 1937, the most outstanding physician and scientists worldwide thought treating hypertension was a crazy idea.

Dr Jon Hay of Liverpool University stated in 1931, "... the greatest danger to a man with a high blood pressure lies in its discovery because then some fool is certain to try and reduce it."

Dr Paul Dudley White, the most renowned Cardiologist of his time, also said in 1937, "... hypertension may be an important compensatory mechanism, which should not be tampered with."

Finally, the author of "Diseases of the Heart," Dr Charles Friedberg, considered 210/100 "mild benign hypertension" and that it "need not be treated."

That brings us to Admiral Ross T. McIntire, an ENT specialist and personal physician to the President of the United States, Franklin Delano Roosevelt.

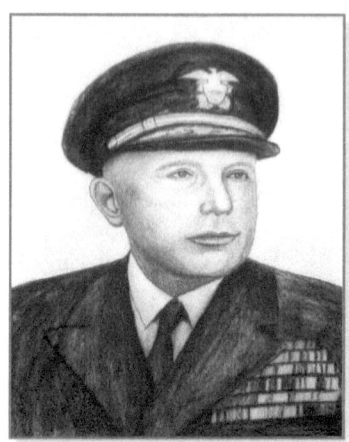

Admiral Ross T. McIntire

Admiral Ross T. McIntire documented the president's blood pressure over several years because he had suffered from hypertension since he was 54.

WASHINGTON. D.C.
April 9 1944

9th	202/102	P.M.	198/98
10th	196/94	"	200/104
11th	192/96	"	204/100
12th	200/102	"	204/96
13th	198/100	"	202/96
14th	206/100	"	200/96
15th	208/102	"	196/100
16th	215/102	"	206/120
17th	210/120	"	206/116 (Dr. Bruen 8th sound)
18th	220/120 (4th sound) Unloop 1 ; kr 8 x t. l. d. ee.
19th	218/120	P.M.	204/104

However, nothing was done about it because it was not considered dangerous, and no proper medications were available.

Eventually, Dr James Paullin of Atlanta, who held the position of President of the American Medical Association, and Dr

Frank Lahey of Boston, founder of the Lahey Clinic in Boston, were consulted to treat the president.

Their recommendations were to reduce the number of hours the President worked daily. They also recommended that he reduce his weight, cut his cigarettes to 10 a day, and reduce the number of cocktails he drinks. The most impactful change was treating the President with Digitalis, a heart medication that does not help blood pressure. Later, the rice diet was the magic prescription for the monumental crisis the United States president faced amid the Second World War.

Some historians believed President Roosevelt had heart failure at the time; whether his poor health at Yalta conference, affected the outcome is debatable. Some historians believe that the president could have taken a stronger stand against controlling Stalin of Eastern Europe.

Churchill's physician, Lord Moran, noted that Roosevelt was "looking straight ahead with his mouth open as if he were not taking things in, and the President appeared ill. I'd give him no more than a few months to live."

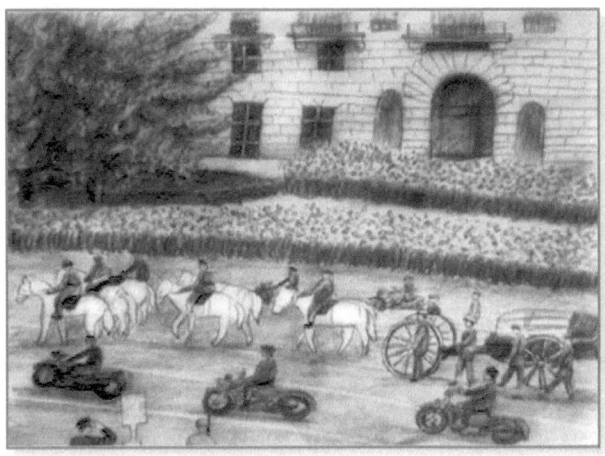

President Roosevelt Funeral

On April 12, 1945, a blood pressure of 300/190 was recorded after Roosevelt reported a severe headache while sitting for a portrait session. He then lost consciousness and died at age 63.

It was reported that Vice President Truman went to see first lady Eleanor who said: "Harry, the president is dead."

He asked if he could do anything for her, to which she replied, "Is there anything we can do for you? For you are the one in trouble now."

Adm Ross T. McIntire, MD, told the nation a few days later that the president's death was unaccepted and not preventable, but was it?

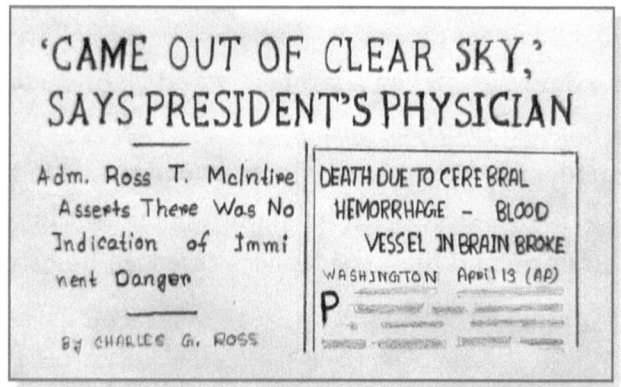

'CAME OUT OF CLEAR SKY,'
SAYS PRESIDENT'S PHYSICIAN

Adm. Ross T. McIntire Asserts There Was No Indication of Immi nent Danger

By CHARLES G. ROSS

DEATH DUE TO CEREBRAL HEMORRHAGE – BLOOD VESSEL IN BRAIN BROKE

WASHINGTON April 13 (AP)

Headline

Influenced by FDR's death, On June 16, 1948, President Harry Truman signed the 'National Heart Act' into law. The US Congress declared, "Whereas the Congress hereby finds and declares that heart and circulation diseases, including high blood pressure, seriously threaten the Nation's health."

"These diseases are the leading cause of death in the United States, and more than one in every three of our people die from them."

The Framingham Heart Study started and continued till the present time.

In an article published in 1970, in the Annals of internal medicine, by Howard Bruenn M, D, FDR's cardiologist, who declared that the president's chart went missing.

Coffee was very well known to have a weak diuretic effect; other plants like digitalis also had a diuretic effect but only in patients with heart failure.

Bloodletting and leeching were used to extract fluid out of the body, not to decrease the body's total fluid, but our grandfathers used them to eliminate the spirits or humor that caused disease.

Dr. Alfred Vogl observed in 1919 while a medical student that the mercury compound used to treat syphilis had a significant diuretic effect and could treat Dropsy or edema.

Mercury compound must be administered by injection and has a significant side effect. As a result of that, it could not be used on a wide scale basis, especially for hypertension.

In 1937, it was realized that sulfonamide antibiotics have a diuretic property. By 1949, Schwarz successfully treated 11 patients with congestive heart failure using sulfonamide.

In the 1950s, four brilliant scientists, James Sprague, Frederick Novello, Karl Beyer, and John Baer, worked for Merck pharmaceutical company. Later, Merck sharp Dohme merged the two companies into the Department of new pharmaceutical discoveries afterwards.

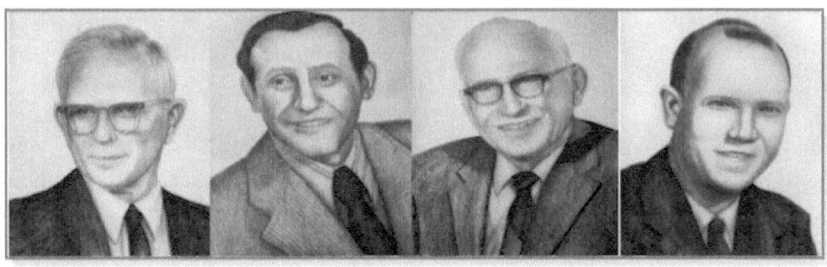

The Merck Sharp & Dohme Group

They used a new method of research called "Design Discovery", where the researchers are looking for a new compound with a specific effect.

Before that Serendipity Played a significant role in pharmaceutical discoveries.

They intended to look for a sulfate compound with a diuretic property, building on the work done by Schwarz and others in the 1940s.

Years later, in 1982, Karl H. Beyer wrote, reflecting on the past:

"In every instance, the important thing was to find the right compound in laboratory animals and to establish acceptance of the utility and safety of the drug in the clinic. If others chose to interpret site and mode of action, or why it lowered blood pressure differently from the thoughts that led to achievement, it mattered little to us."

The Merck Sharp Dohme group synthesized many compounds looking for the one with the most diuretic properties. Chlorothiazide was the compound they sought and found; they called the drug Diuril.

After discovering chlorothiazide, there was an intense internal debate about whether to try it on patients with oedema "Fluid buildup "or hypertension.

In response to the Thalidomide tragedy, when pregnant mothers were prescribed thalidomide for morning sickness, thousands of children were born with congenital disabilities "shortened limbs".

An amendment to the Federal Food, Drug, and Cosmetic Act, called Kefauver-Harris Amendments in 1962, passed congress and became the law which required drug manufacturers to prove the effectiveness and safety of their drug before it was approved.

Hollander and Wilkins 1957, Freis and Wilson 1957, and Tapia et al. 1957 documented that chlorothiazide is a valuable hypotensive agent. Alone and in combination with other hypotensive drugs, it is still valuable.

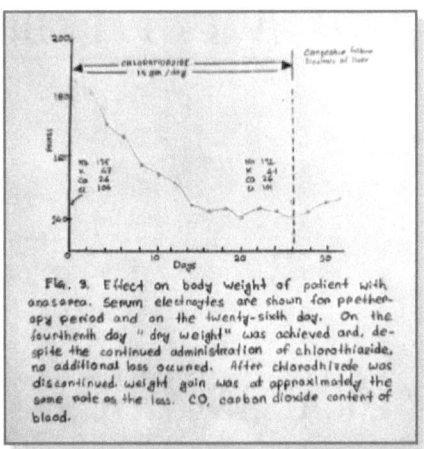

FIG. 3. Effect on body weight of patient with anasarca. Serum electrolytes are shown for pretherapy period and on the twenty-sixth day. On the fourteenth day "dry weight" was achieved and, despite the continued administration of chlorothiazide, no additional loss occurred. After chlorothiazide was discontinued, weight gain was at approximately the same rate as the loss. CO_2 carbon dioxide content of blood.

A landmark randomized and controlled "Veterans Cooperative Study 1964" proved that antihypertensive medication for moderate to severe hypertension was beneficial, with remarkable decreases in death and stroke incidence.

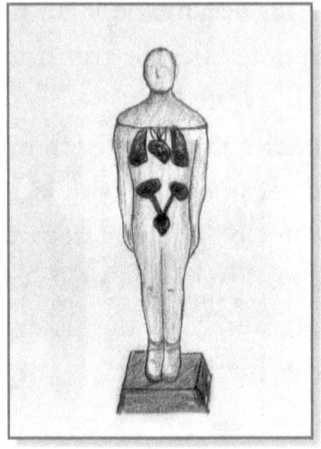

The Diuril Man

CHAPTER 11

LOCAL ANESTHESIA

During the fourth voyage of exploration of the Americas, many Spaniards reported in February 1503 that many locals "never stopped chewing a dry herb ', which was the first recorded description of cocaine reaching Europe.

Europeans consumed coca leaves for the next 250 years, but that consumption never became popular. One of the reasons is that the leaves could not make the trip from South America to Europe without getting rotted.

Later in 1885, a pharmacist chemist from Germany, Friedrich Gaedecke, extracted cocaine from coca leaves.

Soon enough, Angelo Mariana from Corsica mixed wine with coca leaves and made what became a very popular tonic; he named it Vin Mariani; ironically, the alcohol in the wine helped convert the coca leaves into cocaine.

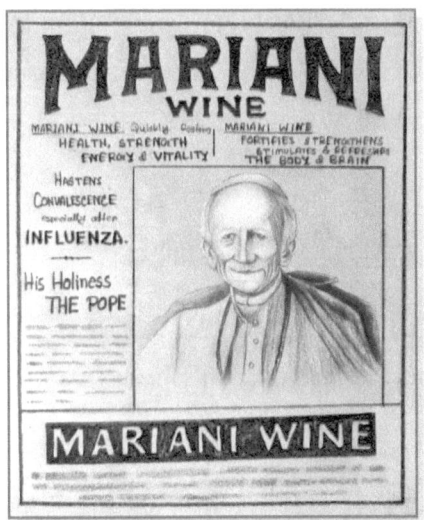

Pop Leo XIII

A wide range of Celebrities used that tonic, including queens, kings, two popes, and many doctors, including Sigmund Freud, who became addicted to cocaine.

As a young man, Sigmund Freud published a book in 1884, the title of which was Uber Coca (about coca}—describing the effects of cocaine on the human body after experimenting on his patients and himself.

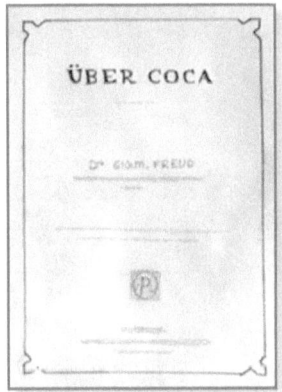

Sigmund Freud's book

At the end of his book 'Uber Coca,' Freud stated that there is a "local application of coca," and this is based on some individual reports which stated that the tongue became numb after tasting cocaine.

Freud claimed that in 1884, he thought of investigating the effect of cocaine on the eye, but he had to delegate that to his friend, Dr Königstein, an "ophthalmic surgeon" who had performed surgery on Freud's father.

The reason Freud left work for his friend was that he had to visit his fiancé, who he had not seen in over two years.

One of his fellow interns and friend in the General Hospital of Vienna was Carl Koller, born in Bohemia (the Czech Republic) and living on the same floor as Freud.

Carl Koller aspired to become an eye surgeon; cataract surgery was a big challenge at that time. This is because of the lack of adequate anesthesia to allow the surgeon to operate without the patient's eye blinking, which would interfere with the surgery.

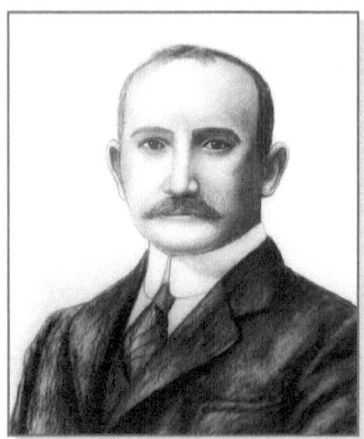

Carl Koller

Dr Königstein never followed through with that research; Carl Koller, who must have been told about the potential local effect of cocaine, took that task immediately. Some historians don't give any credit to Freud, and they claim it was common knowledge that cocaine has a local anesthetic property.

Regardless, Carl Koller made a solution of cocaine leaves, and applied it to one of the eyes of a frog; the other eye was the control,and used a needle to test the sensation of both eyes. In the end, he noted the considerable deference between the two eyes' response to needle stimulation.

Carl Koller could not attend the German Ophthalmological Society Meeting in Heidelberg during the fall of 1884 because of his poor finances. He then asked his friend Dr Josef Brettauer to present the findings and demonstrate the local anesthetic effect of cocaine on the eye of a large dog. The response to the presentation and the finding was extraordinary.

The fact that Freud missed discovering the local effect of cocaine created a controversy, as Freud's reaction changed over time.

Initially, he was jealous of Cael Koller, but as time passed, that feeling faded, and in one of his letters, he called Carl (Coca Koller).

In January 1885, Dr Fritz Zinner was a colleague of Koller at the General University Hospital of Vienna. During an argument, he called Koller an Impudent Jew, so Koller slapped Zinner in the face.

A duel with swords, which was illegal then, occurred in Vienna; Zinner was wounded, and Koller was not harmed.

Koller's chances to practice and advance in academia dwindled to the point that he left Vienna and ended up in New York in 1888.

The interest in discovering safer and non-addictive local anesthetics grew as cocaine use became widespread.

Starting in 1892, a chemist from Munich, Germany, named Albert Einhorn started working on a substitute for cocaine; his efforts were unsuccessful despite many attempts.

Einhorn never gave up, and finally, in 1905, Novocain was verified by the notorious Heinrich Braun to be more effective and less toxic than cocaine. Although Einhom hoped it would be used on wounded soldiers, physicians preferred general anesthesia for amputation; however, Novocain became very popular among dentists and became a household name. Surprisingly the name is still commonly used, even though Novocain is not being used at all.

In 1955, Senator John Kennedy had multiple back surgeries, followed by significant compilations, and his surgeon recommended that the senator should consult a physician in New York called Janet Travell.

Janet Travell was a trained cardiologist but had changed her interests and started treating patients for chronic pain at her father's office,who was a general practitioner.

Dr Travell described how the senator in May 1955 "could barely navigate the 3 or 4 steps down from the curb to the front door, below street level."

She used local Novocain to treat Senator Kennedy's chronic pain. She also discovered that Kennedy's left leg was ¾ of an inch shorter than the right leg, so she recommended a unique shoe to help his pain.

Finally, Dr Travell recommended that Senator Kennedy use a rocking chair, so Kennedy bought an old-fashioned rocker for $24.95, about $100 today's money, which became a signature of his presidency.

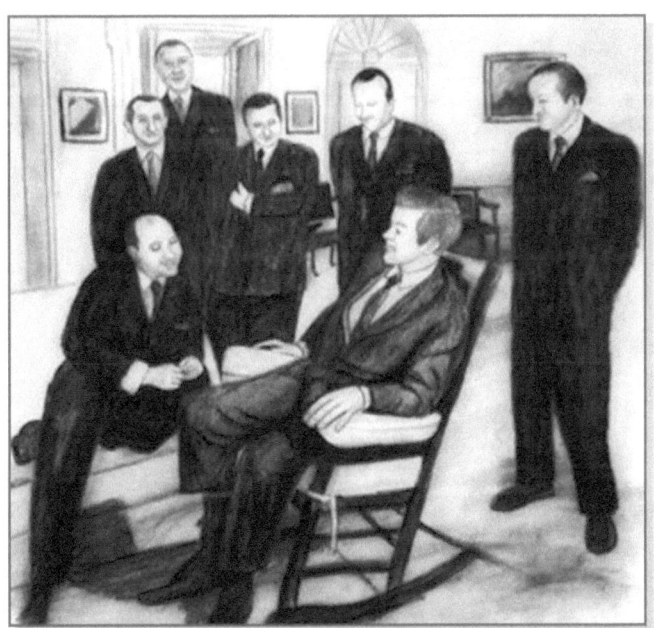

President Kennedy's rocking chair

Many historians believe that Novocain helped Kennedy secure the presidency since his core message was centered around his youth, vigor and energy, which would not have been possible to project without Dr Travell's treatments.

A Los Angeles Times editorial stated: "Unlike Franklin Roosevelt's concealment of his polio, Kennedy's pretended vigor was not a defensive maneuver.... [It] was the core of his message."

The Novocain's treatments must have had a favorable effect on the senator as the treatment continued for years. Also, he named Dr Travell as his physician once he was elected president of the United States to become the first women to occupy that position, despite her being a registered Republican, and she was treating his rival senator Goldwater.

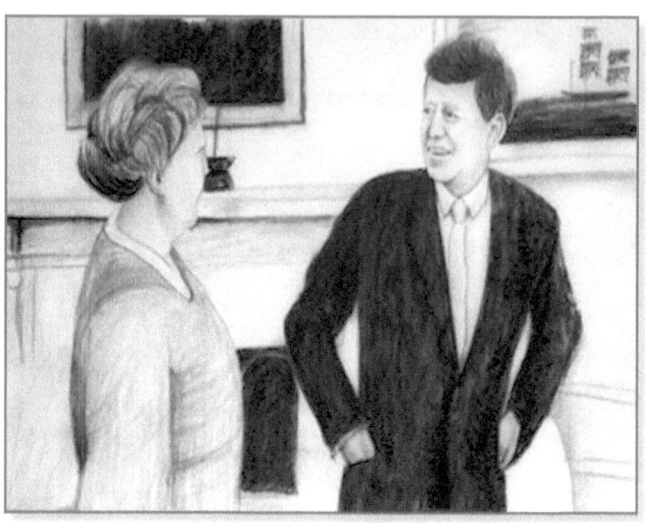

Kennedy wrote, "For Dr Travell-Who made the smile possible-"

A new use of Novocain became prevalent in late 1950; it was marketed as a "fountain of youth drug" until it was banned by the FDA in 1982. In the past few years, that drug is making a comeback in popularity, thanks for the internet marketing.

Under communist Romania in 1952, Ana Aslan, a physician, claimed that her medication, which she named Gerovital H3, was a miracle drug that rejuvenated the body and mind. The main ingredient in that medicine is nothing but Novocain.

According to Romanian officials, over 12 000 people, including presidents and other celebrities, visit Romania annually to try that drug.

Upon using Novocain, it was found that its local anesthetic effect is short-lived, and a significant percentage of patients developed an allergy to the product, so the race began to find a substitute.

It was well known that the Giant Reed, a tall perennial plant, produces a toxic substance, Gramine, that kills animals and insects. To study its potential as a pesticide, interests developed in synthesizing Gramine.

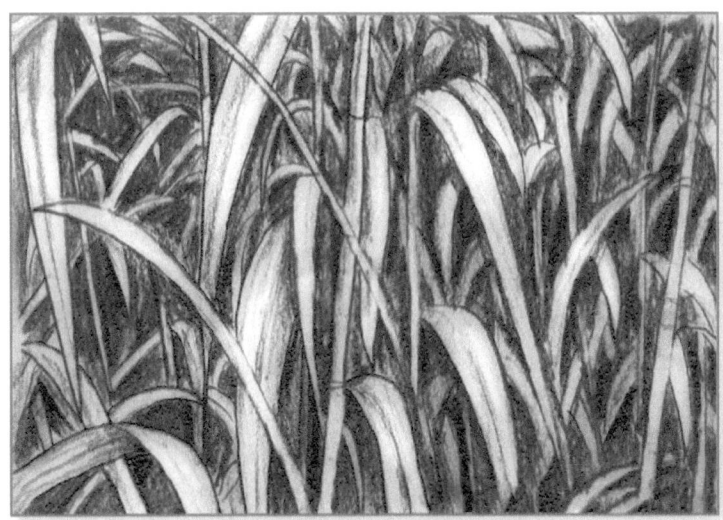

Giant Reed

Holger Erdtman, a Swedish postdoctoral student in 1934, was given the task of synthesizing Gramine; unfortunately, or fortunately, he failed to synthesize Gramine; instead, he produced another substance similar in structure to Gramine but has different properties (Isomer). It was customary for him to taste all the new products he produced in the lab, and to his surprise, this one numbed his tongue and lips.

In 1935, Nils Lofgren joined Erdtmen in his quest to produce a local anesthetic better than Novocain with a small grant from Astra, a small Swedish pharmaceutical company.

The results of sixteen substances were produced and sent to Astra for testing, which was conducted by Ulf von Euler, a more objective method than tasting the material.

He compared this substance's effect on the cornea of a rabbit upon irritating the cornea with a hair and monitored the blinking that followed, and he found that all these substances were not better than Novocain.

All interests and funding dried out. However, years later, Nils Lofgren, who has never given up, started experimenting with material from where he fell off; with the help of a young chemist Bengt Lundqvist, they produced many new substances.

Among these substances, two stood out, LL 30, and LL 31, named after the initials of both discoverers, and the number stood for the discovery sequence.

The tasting was not an objective way to measure the new product's efficacy against Novocain, the most popular local anesthetic at the time. They did not, however, have enough funding to purchase rabbits for laboratory experiments.

Bengt Lundqvist convinced Nils Lofgren to allow him to experiment with the LL 30 on himself; despite Lindqvist's lack of knowledge and experience, he started experimenting on himself, using a borrowed anesthesia book as a guide.

He injected himself at different sites and recorded the onset and duration of the anesthetic effect, as well as his blood pressure and heart rate.

They quickly applied for a patent for LL 30 under the name Lidocaine, which was granted in July 1943; they approached different drug companies for a sponsor. After one rejection, they obtained Astra's support. Astra was a small Swedish pharmaceutical company at that time.

On the train trip to meet the executive at Aster, Lundqvist remembered that he did not inject LL 30 in the Jaw and had no data for that. He injected himself while on the train, and became unable to speak, with visible drooling because of the anesthetic effect, which made Astra more receptive to adopting lidocaine.

Dr Torsten Gordh, the only formally trained anesthesiologist in Sweden then, was asked to verify the efficacy and test the safety of lidocaine. The trials started in 1944 and lasted three years.

Dr Gordh tested it on his colleagues, students, and patients. He paid the patients five Swedish crowns each (about a dollar), and his students were given a pack of American cigarettes; it is unknown if he paid his colleagues.

Both Lundqvist and Lofgren became very rich, and due to taxes in Sweden, Lundqvist bought a sailing boat and died while diving, trying to fix his boat.

Lofgren moved to Switzerland to avoid paying taxes but returned later to Sweden and affected by depression with alcoholism; he committed suicide.

Xylocaine was approved in the United States in late 1948, and soon after that, the Department of Defense ordered 10 million doses of Xylocaine to be used in the Korean War.

However, shortly after that, the Pentagon cancelled the order because the officials at the Pentagon were not convinced it was better than Novocain, to justify such a higher price.

The pharmaceutical company's representative in Washington convinced the officer in charge to try some of the lidocaine ointment on his tongue. The officer could not talk correctly, that made the Pentagon reinstate the order.

CHAPTER 12

VACCINATION

Lady Mary Wortley Montagu, the wife of the British ambassador to the ottoman empire, witnessed firsthand the procedure of variolation (introducing a small amount of the infected material to healthy people). This was done in Istanbul to protect the healthy from contracting Smallpox, and when she returned to London in 1718, she introduced it to the British public.

The public was not receptive to such a procedure, so it was first applied to convicted prisoners who would be freed if they survived. Later, Lady Mary Wortley Montagu ended up with subjecting her children to variolation.

Patrick Russell was another observer of the practice of variolation in Aleppo, Syria, which was part of the ottoman empire at that time, and in 1771 reported another way to prevent small box infection, by breathing through vinegar-soaked cloth.

In 1796, a maid, Sarah Nelmes, consulted Dr Edward Jenner

regarding a rash on her hand. Jenner recognized that she was suffering from Cowpox, and under questioning, Mrs Nelmes told Dr Jenner that she had been milking a cow with a similar spot on its Udder (breast).

It was well known that some people could not be inoculated, even though they were never infected with smallpox. But rather, they had been infected with cowpox before.

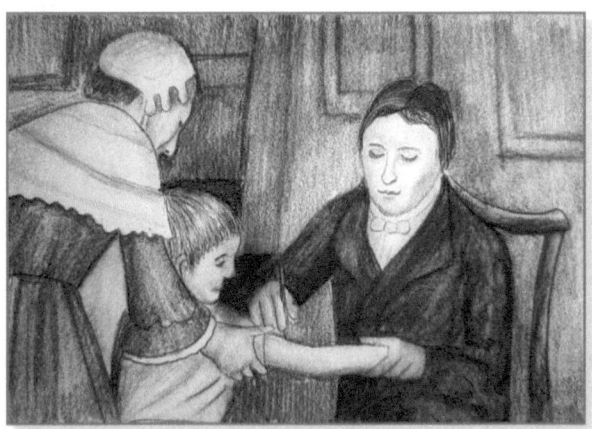

Dr Edward Jenner

Dr Jenner took the next step and tried using scrap from Cowpox's infected patient to inject into a healthy person, to find out if any that would provide any protection.

He chose poor James Phipps, an eight-year boy, the son of his gardener, "Informed consent" needs not to be bothered with especially if the subject is poor, and his father worked for the scientist.

The boy became mildly sick with Cowpox but recovered in a few days.

Dr Jenner did not stop there but went on to infect the boy with the actual smallpox virus, Luckily, the boy did not get sick, and Dr Jenner concluded that his experiment was successful and called his procedure Vaccination after the Latin name of the Cow "Vacca."

In 1940, the USA was on the verge of being dragged into war in Europe.

The leadership of the army's biggest fear was to repeat the first war's disastrous experience, as more soldiers died from the flu than from fighting in battle.

So, Henry L. Stimson, the U.S. secretary of war, formed a board of experts to find a physician to lead the effort to prevent an outbreak of influenza among the soldiers.

They chose Dr Thomas Francis, who had worked with the flu virus for some time. After working for ten years at the Rockefeller Institute in New York, he moved to Ann Arbor to start a new department for preventing epidemic diseases at the University of Michigan.

Dr Francis's choice for an assistant was the young Jonas Salk, the future inventor of the polio vaccine.

They agreed that a killed virus would stimulate the immune system to produce protection against the disease, and they went to work on modifying the Flu virus to make the vaccine.

After over a year, they were ready for trial, which involved giving the vaccine to many people and comparing their immunity against the flu with the immunity of an equal number of people who were not given the vaccine.

They chose two state hospitals for the mentally ill to conduct their trial on these residents; DRs Francis and Salk injected 8000 poor men with the new vaccine or a placebo without proper consent.

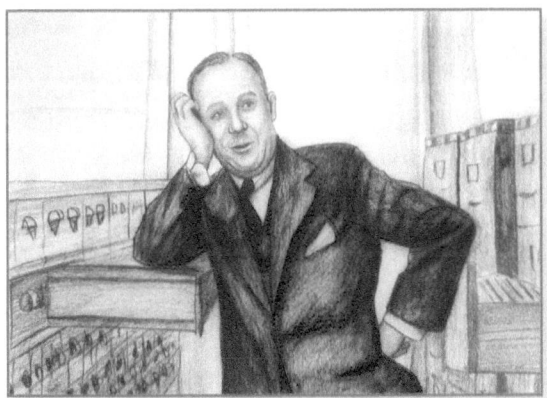
Dr Thomas Francis

Luckily, none of the mentally ill, who received the vaccine, became seriously ill.

Drs Francis and Salk found that the antibody to counter the flu rose 85 % above the baseline level in those who received the vaccine. It is not so with the other patient who got the placebo.

Unfortunately, for Drs Francis and Salk, there was no influenza epidemic that year and the trial did not fully answer whether the vaccine effectively prevented the Flu.

The next step, in the following year, was a more outrageous experiment by today's standards than their first on the 8000 mentally ill subjects.

This is because they intentionally infected a number of the patients who had received the vaccine with the live Flu virus by spraying a mist of infected tissue into the patient's nostrils.

Only 16 percent developed the flu out of the vaccinated individuals, while nearly half of non-vaccinated got sick with the Flu.

Conflict and fissure developed between the mentor, Dr Fisher, and his protégée, Dr Salk. This occurred when it was discovered that, Salk had struck a deal with one of the pharmaceutical companies, Park Davis, to provide the company with all information regarding vaccine developments in return for 100 dollars monthly consultant fee, industrial espionage by today's standard.

On the other hand, Salk was suspicious of his Mentor's intention because of what Dr fisher had written about him.

"Dr Salk is a member of the Jewish race but has, I believe, a very great capacity to get on with people."

Despite recent cases in New York state in 2022, Polio remains a disease of the past, and not on the mind of most people, except during the routine visit to pediatricians for vaccinating children.

Polio was known to the ancient Egyptians, as demonstrated in the following picture:

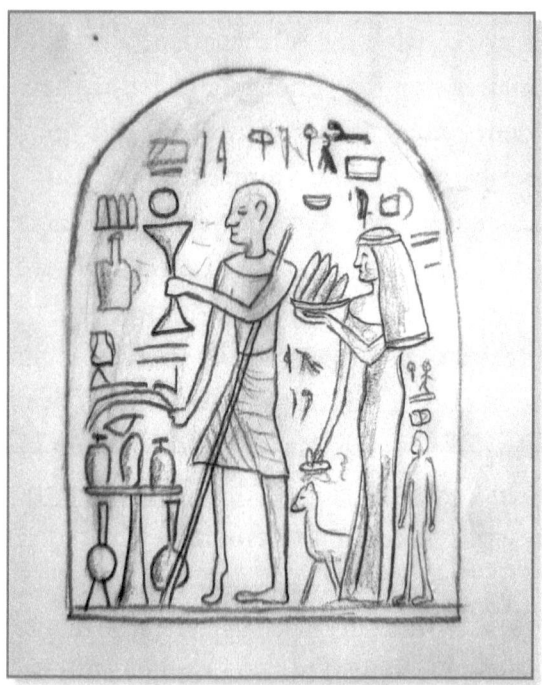

An ancient man with polio

It did not become a major source of concern in the US until the 19th century and later when three epidemics hit the United States in 1916, 1946, and 1949.

In 1921 Franklin D Roosevelt, the future president was diagnosed with Paralic Polio. He was 39 years old and was paralyzed from the waist down.

Franklin D Roosevelt founded the National Foundation for Infantile Paralysis, NFIP, in 1938. This is intended to help victims of the disease and fund researchers in their fight against Polio.

The financial support from the foundation was crucial in developing the polio vaccine. The foundation donated $ 150000 in the first year for researching the Polio vaccine, while the federal government spending on polio research was $ 75000 for the same year.

In 1934, two separate groups of scientists, John Kolmer of Temple University in Philadelphia and Brodie of New York University Medical College, conducted experiments on two different polio vaccines on humans, they used orphans as test subjects. with disastrous results. That led Eleanor Roosevelt to request an investigation by the Surgeon General's office.

In 1947, Dr Jonas Salk, after working in Ann Arbor on the Flu vaccine, wanted to have a lab of his own, and he moved to the University of Pittsburg. The existing lab was, however, small and insufficient to conduct any meaningful research.

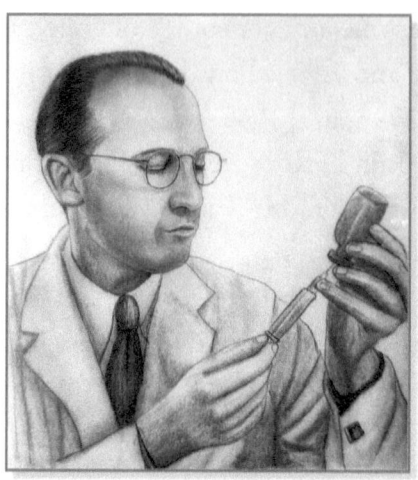

Dr Jonas Salk

Promising to work on a vaccine for polio, he attracted significant donations from the non-profit organization National Foundation for Infantile Paralysis.

Before Salk, there were significant advances in the knowledge about the Polio virus, from the port of entry to the serum phase, the three different kinds of polioviruses, and the ability to grow the virus in tissue.

With financial support again from the National Foundation for Infantile Paralysis, between 1945 and 1949, five years before Dr Salk's discovery, a brilliant virologist (a scientist work with viruses) at John Hopkins, Isabel Morgan (1911 – 1996) was able to immunize monkey with a killed Polio virus.

However, in 1949, she suddenly resigned from her position to be a housewife to care for her stepson, who had a learning disability. Millions of women in the United States and around the world still experience the phenomenon of women leaving or downgrading their careers for family's sake.

Using Live viruses to make vaccines was the standard in the 1940s. However, Dr Jonas Salk's experience with the neutralized (killed) flu vaccine under Dr Thomas Francis in Ann Arbor made him choose this method to produce the Polio vaccine.

His research was painful, costly, and slow. Finally, he produced an inactive (neutralized) Poliovirus using formaldehyde, a chemical used as a disinfectant in funeral homes and medical labs.

First, he tested his vaccine on monkeys, and it was successful. Next, he had to conduct a risky experiment by testing it on humans.

In 1952, he injected the neutralized virus into children with Polio. He reasoned that first, they have some immunity from the disease, and second if they ended up being infected, the damage would be limited compared to the potential damage to a healthy child. What a justification.

The antibody against polio was used to prove efficacy, and his experiment worked.

Next, he inoculated sixty-three mentally institutionalized disabled children at the Polk State School in Pittsburg, an unacceptable practice by today's standards.

Dr Salk also gave his inactive virus to disabled children from diseases other than Polio, again thinking that if they ended up infected, the residual damage would be less than the damage to a healthy child, and it worked.

The moral and ethical justification of these experiments is, at best, questionable by today's standard; the informed consent could not have been more flawed.

However, in Dr Salk's defense, his next step was to inject himself, his wife, and his three children with the inactive virus, a practice carried over from the nineteenth century.

On 23 January 1953, Dr Salk announced his results on 161 children who received his "Killed Vaccine," asking for support from the scientific advisory committee and the National Foundation for Infantile Paralysis.

Despite significant opposition, this is the justification put forward by the leadership of the National Foundation for Infantile Paralysis:

.. If [we wait until more] research is carried out, large numbers of human beings will develop poliomyelitis who might have been prevented from doing so."

It was a convincing argument, which led to the approval of a much larger study of the Salk vaccine. Later, the foundation appointed Dr Thomas Francis of Ann Arbor, the inventor of the Flu vaccine and the prior boss of Dr Salk, to be the head of the expert group overseeing the study.

On April 12, 1955, Dr Thomas Francis rereleased the study result of over 1.8 million children vaccinated with the Salk vaccine, which was 80-90 % effective.

Ten days after the approval of the vaccine, a tragedy struck. Thousands of Polio cases were reported, 260 children were paralyzed, and 11 died right after vaccination. All infected were traced back to one manufacturer in Berkley, California.

This became what is known as the Cutter incident, named after the Cutter laboratory, one of the six companies entrusted to manufacture the vaccine in 1955.

It turned out that a year earlier, in 1954, in the NIH, Dr Bernice Eddy, a scientist, discovered that the samples submitted from the cutter laboratory for approval before manufacturing were contaminated with live Polio virus. Those samples made injected monkeys sick and some paralyzed.

Dr Eddy alerted her superior, but for an unknown reason,

she was ignored. One could not help but speculate that her gender played a role in silencing her.

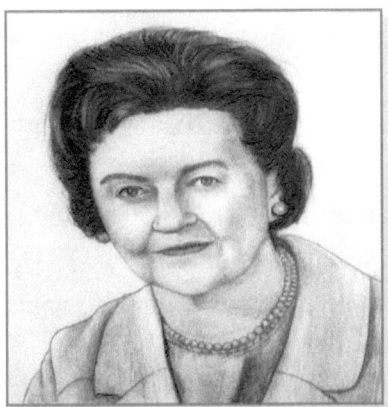

Dr Bernice Eddy "silenced whistleblower."

The Cutter incident led to the resignation of the U.S. Secretary of Health, Education and Welfare and the head of the NIH.

Those resignations did not regain the general public's confidence in the United States and worldwide. However, the marked decrease in the incidences of Polio in states and countries where the Cutter vaccine was not used, and without any incident of paralytic Polio in the vaccinated children, convinced the majority of the public that the vaccine is safe and effective.

In 1955, Dr Jonas Salk was asked about the decision not to patent the vaccine, and his response was unaccepted:

"Well, the people, I would say. There is no patent. Could you patent the sun?"

Because of the overwhelming demands, and limited supplies, a black market developed, and the Have-Nots could not receive the vaccine for a while.

The Cutter laboratory was found not liable for the dreadful

incident because the government signed off on the manufacturing of the vaccine, but it was ordered to pay a fine of $139,000 for false advertising that its vaccine was safe.

Albert Bruce Sabin was born Abram Saperstejn in 1906, and he immigrated with his family to New York at the age of 12 from Biatystok, a part of Russia at the time; now, it is a Polish city.

Dr Sabin became interested in studying Polio right after graduation from New York University in 1931, influenced by his mentor. He became instrumental in the valuable and essential Polio virus disease process knowledge.

Dr Sabin examined hundreds of autopsies from Polio victims and found that plenty of Polio Viruses were in the GI tract. Only a few in the nasopharyngeal proved that the port of entry of the polio virus was the stomach and intestine.

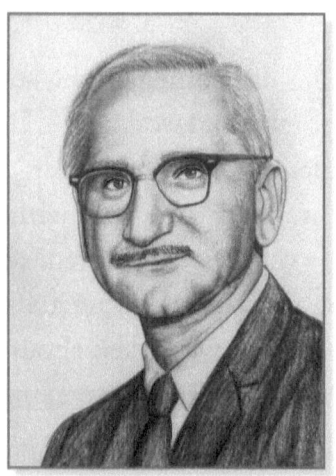

Dr Albert Sabin

He discovered a procedure to weaken the Polio virus and used it as a vaccine by mouth. Working for the Lederle Laboratories in New York,

Dr Sabin tested his oral and attenuated (weakened) vaccine on thousands of monkeys, later he tested it on 30 adult volunteers recruited from the inmates of the federal prison of Chillicothe in Ohio, and as it was customary on his daughter and himself.

As outlined in a letter, those volunteers received an honorarium of $ 25 and three free days. Dr Sabin send a check for $1175 to cover the cost to the federal reformatory.

Despite his success, Dr Sabin was not granted permission to conduct a more extensive study in the US, similar to the Salk vaccine study, because the US government was already committed to the Salk vaccine, and because of the Cutter incident, the public could not tolerate another new study.

In January of 1956, a Soviet health delegation was touring the United States; their main target was obtaining the Salk vaccine technology. However, they requested to visit Dr Sabin to learn about his new oral Vaccine.

The Soviet delegation was required to travel by train only, and an American observer closely monitored the delegation; it was thought that at least one of the delegation members was a KGB officer.

The Soviet Union invited Dr Salk and Dr Sabin to visit Moscow. Dr Salk declined, but Dr Sabin was happy to visit to promote his oral vaccine. He was given permission after two intensive FBI interviews, because there was a concern in the US government that the samples he would give to the Soviets could be used as a biological weapon.

Dr Sabin's argument to the Soviet scientist favoring his oral vaccine over Dr Salk's injectable vaccine included that it could be given by mouth. That is, it requires a single dose instead of the three doses of Dr Salk's vaccine, the immunity is more durable.

That it produces passive immunization, that would happen when the vaccinated person sheds some of the attenuated vaccine (weakened) through their body excretion, which in turn would immunize the non-vaccinated member of the community.

Over 77 million people were vaccinated in the Soviet Union using the oral Sabin vaccine. The strongly positive result of safety and effectiveness was announced, but doubt circulated among many in the conference held in Washington DC in June 1959

A member of the Soviet delegation remarked:

"I would like to assure [you] of one thing, that we in the Soviet Union love our children and are as concerned for their wellbeing as much as people in the United States, or any other part of the world are for their children."

To give the Soviet study credibility, The World Health Organization sent a Yale virologist to Moscow to review the trial; her report was affirmative.

The Soviets promoted the vaccine as their own, and it was called "the communist vaccine."

As with Dr Jonas Salk, Dr Albert Sabin refused to patent his vaccine to keep the vaccine price as low as possible.

In 2012, Forbes magazine estimated that Salk would have made 2.5 billion dollars and Sabin would have made 6 billion dollars if they had patented their vaccines.

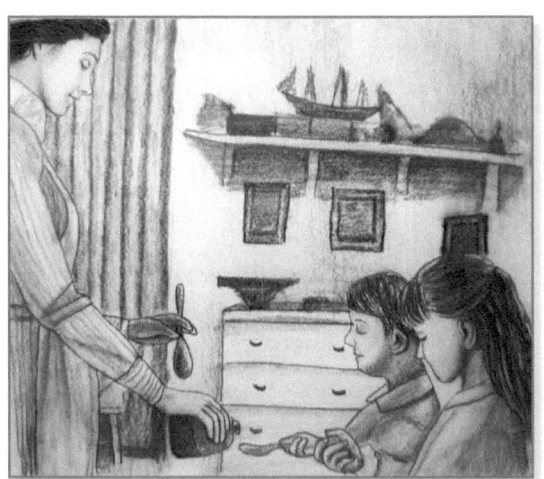

Mary Poppin

Since the oral vaccine was being given with some sugar, it inspired the song: "a spoonful of sugar makes the medicine go down."